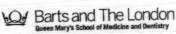

Oxford University Press makes no representation, express or implied, that the drug dosages in this book are correct. Readers must therefore always check the product information and clinical procedures with the most up-to-date published product information and data sheets provided by the manufacturers and the most recent codes of conduct and safety regulations. The authors and the publishers do not accept responsibility or legal liability for any errors in the text or for the misuse or misapplication of material in this work.

► Except where otherwise stated, drug doses and recommendations are for the non-pregnant adult who is not breast-feeding.

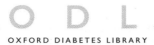

OXFORD DIABETES LIBRARY

Insulin Pump Therapy and Continuous Glucose Monitoring

Edited by

John Pickup

Professor of Diabetes and Metabolism,
King's College London School of Medicine,
Guy's Hospital, London SE1 9RT, UK

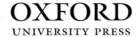

OXFORD
UNIVERSITY PRESS

OXFORD
UNIVERSITY PRESS

Great Clarendon Street, Oxford OX2 6DP

Oxford University Press is a department of the University of Oxford.
It furthers the University's objective of excellence in research, scholarship,
and education by publishing worldwide in

Oxford New York

Auckland Cape Town Dar es Salaam Hong Kong Karachi
Kuala Lumpur Madrid Melbourne Mexico City Nairobi
New Delhi Shanghai Taipei Toronto

With offices in

Argentina Austria Brazil Chile Czech Republic France Greece
Guatemala Hungary Italy Japan Poland Portugal Singapore
South Korea Switzerland Thailand Turkey Ukraine Vietnam

Oxford is a registered trade mark of Oxford University Press
in the UK and in certain other countries

Published in the United States
by Oxford University Press Inc., New York

© Oxford University Press, 2009

The moral rights of the author(s) have been asserted
Database right Oxford University Press (maker)

First published 2009

British Library Cataloguing in Publication Data

Data available

Library of Congress Cataloging in Publication Data

Data available

Typeset by Newgen Imaging Systems (P) Ltd., Chennai, India
Printed in Great Britain
on acid-free paper by
Ashford Colour Press Ltd., Gosport, Hampshire.

ISBN 978-0-19-956860-4

10 9 8 7 6 5 4 3 2 1

Contents

Abbreviations list

BG	blood glucose
CGM	continuous glucose monitoring
CIPII	continuous intraperitoneal insulin infusion
CIT	conventional insulin injection therapy
CSII	continuous subcutaneous insulin infusion
CT	computer tomography
CVD	cardiovascular disease
DCCT	diabetes control and complications trial
DKA	diabetic ketoacidosis
GI	glycaemic index
HbA$_{1c}$	haemoglobin A$_{1c}$
HbF	fetal haemoglobin
I:C	insulin:carbohydrate ratio
ICER	incremental cost-effectiveness ratio
IP	intraperitoneal
ISF	insulin sensitivity factor
LED	light-emitting diodes
MDI	multiple daily insulin injections
MRI	magnetic resonance imaging
NS	not significant
OAD	oral antidiabetic agents
QALY	quality adjusted life year
QoL	quality of life
RCT	randomized controlled trials
RR	rate ratio
RT-CGM	real-time continuous glucose monitoring
TDD	total daily dose

Contributors

Tadej Battelino
Professor, Department of
Paediatric Endocrinology,
Diabetes and Metabolism, UMC—
University Children's Hospital,
University of Ljubljana, Slovenia

Peter Hammond
Consultant Diabetologist,
Harrogate District Hospital,
Harrogate, UK

Hélène Hanaire
Professor, Department
of Diabetology,
Metabolic Diseases and Nutrition,
University Hospital Toulouse,
France

Lutz Heinemann
Partner and Consultant,
Profil Institut für
Stoffwechselforschung GmbH,
Neusse, Germany

Julia Kidd
Diabetes Specialist Nurse, Guy's
and St Thomas's Hospitals NHS
Foundation Trust, Guy's Hospital,
London, UK

Siobhan Pender
Diabetes Specialist Nurse,
Guy's and St Thomas's
Hospitals NHS Foundation
Trust, Guy's Hospital,
London, UK

John Pickup
Professor of Diabetes
and Metabolism,
King's College London
School of Medicine, Guy's
Hospital, London, UK

Howard Wolpert
Director, Insulin Pump Program,
Joslin Diabetes Center,
Boston, USA

Nardos Yemane
Dietician,
Guy's and St Thomas's
Hospitals NHS Foundation Trust,
Guy's Hospital, London, UK

Chapter 1

Insulin pump therapy: then and now

John Pickup

Key points

- Continuous subcutaneous insulin infusion (CSII) is also known as insulin pump therapy
- CSII is a form of intensified insulin treatment, mostly used for selected patients with type 1 diabetes
- Insulin pump therapy was originally developed as a research tool, but is now part of routine clinical practice
- In CSII, short-acting (monomeric) insulin is infused subcutaneously at variable rates (basal and prandial) from a portable infusion pump
- The main clinical indications are frequent and disabling hypoglycaemia and/or a continued elevated HbA_{1c} in spite of best attempts with insulin injection therapy (usually multiple daily insulin injections, MDI)

Continuous subcutaneous insulin infusion (CSII), popularly known as insulin pump therapy, is a form of intensified insulin treatment for people with diabetes, with the strongest evidence base for its effectiveness in type 1 diabetes. In CSII, strict glycaemic control is achieved by infusing short-acting insulin subcutaneously at variable rates using a portable infusion pump, usually worn around the waist.

1.1 The history and rationale of insulin pump therapy

CSII was first developed and used in the 1970s as a research procedure, though it has now become a routine form of treatment for selected people with type 1 diabetes. Its use in type 2 diabetes is currently being explored (see Chapter 7).

Thirty years ago, at the time insulin pump therapy was first used, it was uncertain whether the microvascular complications of diabetes are an intrinsic part of the diabetic process, developing in parallel with diabetes, or are direct results of prolonged hyperglycaemia damaging the small blood vessels. However, treatment methods at the time were unable to maintain near normoglycaemia for long enough to test experimentally the link between poor control and the tissue complications. Several organizations therefore called for the development of more physiological methods of insulin delivery that might dramatically improve metabolic control (Cahill *et al.* 1976).

The rationale for using insulin infusion instead of injections and the concept of physiological insulin administration arise from the notion that mimicking the insulin delivery of the healthy person will markedly improve metabolic control in diabetes (Figure 1.1). Physiological insulin delivery has three main components: a slow and constant delivery throughout 24 hours (the basal insulin), boosts at mealtimes (the prandial insulin), and feedback (closed-loop) control, with the pancreatic islets sensing glucose and altering insulin secretion so as to maintain euglycaemia.

Attempts to construct an 'artificial endocrine pancreas' with closed-loop insulin delivery had been under development since the 1960s (Kadish 1963) and by the mid 1970s researchers had developed a large and fairly complex bedside apparatus for feedback-controlled insulin administration, operating over a day or so. This pumped venous blood from the diabetic patient to the device, where blood glucose

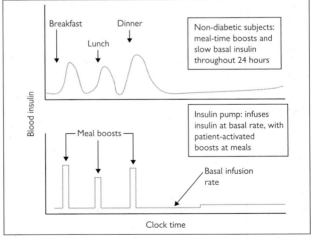

Figure 1.1 Blood insulin concentrations in a healthy individual (upper panel) and how CSII mimics the physiological insulin profiles by infusing insulin at a variable basal rate with boosts at mealtimes (lower panel).

concentrations were measured and insulin or glucose pumped back into the bloodstream according to algorithms (rules), relating glucose to the insulin infusion rate needed to maintain normoglycaemia (Albisser et al. 1974; Pfeiffer et al. 1974).

However, this was clearly not a technology that could be applied to everyday diabetes care, and consideration was given to whether almost as good control could be achieved without closing-the-loop—just by infusing insulin at preset basal and prandial rates according to the patient's needs. This is called 'open-loop' insulin infusion.

In a pioneering study in Paris by Slama et al. (1974), seven people with type 1 diabetes were infused intravenously with regular insulin for 1–5 days, using a peristaltic pump worn in a shoulder bag. With a basal rate and 15-fold augmentation at mealtimes, very good glycaemic control was achieved by this simple open-loop system. Extending this notion, and arguing that longer periods of infusion would be possible without the potential dangers of thrombosis and septicaemia associated with the intravenous route, we started investigating variable-rate subcutaneous insulin as an approach to achieving strict glycaemic control in type 1 diabetes. The first full paper in 1978, studied 12 subjects with type 1 diabetes in a hospital setting using CSII for a day or so (Pickup et al. 1978). A portable battery-driven syringe pump weighing 159g (the 'Mill Hill Infuser'), which was originally developed for drug infusion studies in animals, was adapted to deliver at two rates: a basal and an 8-fold higher rate for 17min which the patient engaged before meals. Short-acting, monocomponent pork insulin was infused from the pump via a fine nylon catheter, with the end implanted in the subcutaneous tissue.

The results of this early study were encouraging, the mean blood glucose level being reduced after just 1 day in 8 out of 12 subjects from 9.7 ± 3.8mmol/L during conventional insulin injection treatment to 5.2 ± 1.3mmol/L (p < 0.01) during insulin pump therapy. The efficacy of CSII was quickly confirmed by other groups (Tamborlane et al. 1979a; Champion et al. 1980) and numerous trials then followed in which control was improved and optimized on CSII and the extended outpatient use and safety of CSII was explored (Pickup et al. 1979b; Mecklenburg et al. 1982).

Several early studies showed that the good glycaemic control that is possible with CSII is also accompanied by a return towards normal blood levels of many intermediary metabolites that are usually disordered on injection therapy, including lactate, ketones, lipids, and amino acids (Pickup et al. 1979a; Tamborlane et al. 1979b). This finding was important in showing that these metabolic abnormalities are secondary to suboptimal insulin replacement in diabetes.

1.2 **Some landmark clinical trials using insulin pump therapy**

As originally intended, CSII has indeed been used in many clinical trials in which the effects of pump-induced near normoglycaemia on the course of microvascular disease in type 1 diabetes was compared to the poor control of conventional insulin injection therapy. Some notable randomized controlled trials of control and complications were the Kroc Study involving five centres in the United Kingdom and North America (Kroc Collaborative Study Group 1984); the Steno Study in Copenhagen, Denmark (Steno Study Group 1982); the Oslo Study in Norway (Dahl-Jørgensen *et al.* 1986); and the Diabetes Control and Complications Trial (DCCT) (Diabetes Control and Complications Trial Research Group 1993). Although subjects in the DCCT were randomized to conventional or intensive treatment, they were allowed to choose whether the intensive therapy was via multiple daily insulin injections (MDI) or CSII, and over the mean study duration of 6.5 years, 124 patients used CSII for >90% of the time, and 284 used MDI (the rest used both CSII and MDI). The mean HbA$_{1c}$ was about 0.2%–0.4% lower on CSII than MDI.

1.3 **The technology of CSII in brief (see Chapter 3)**

Most current insulin infusion pumps are still battery-operated syringe drivers (similar to the first CSII pump) and have a motor-driven lead screw which advances an actuator in engagement with the plunger of the syringe. Short-acting insulin (monomeric insulin is now the recommended pump insulin) is infused from the pump reservoir via a plastic cannula which terminates in either a fine-gauge needle or flexible catheter implanted in the subcutaneous tissue (see Chapter 3). The basal insulin infusion rates are altered electronically by depressing keys or buttons on the pump and can be preset to automatically change at any time in the day; for example, a lower nocturnal rate to avoid hypoglycaemia, an augmented pre-breakfast rate to reduce the dawn phenomenon, and a variable daytime rate, according to requirements and activities. Temporary basal rates lasting for a few hours can be used, say for less insulin during and after exercise.

Mealtime insulin boosts are activated by the patient by keying in the required amount according to the size and composition of the meal. More sophisticated prandial insulin profiling is possible for special circumstances, for example, by delivery of extended square waves for high fat/protein meals or anticipated delayed absorption and dual waves (standard plus extended) for high carbohydrate/high fat meals. Pumps now have bolus calculators that estimate and advise on the required mealtime insulin, based on the patient entering the carbohydrate content of the meal and (depending on the pump) such other factors as the most recent blood glucose level and the insulin sensitivity, and taking into account the insulin 'on board' (i.e. the amount remaining from the previous bolus).

Alarm and safety features usually include alerts for occlusion, over-delivery, and near-empty reservoir, amongst other events. Pump data can now be downloaded to a personal computer or web-based software.

Alternative pump technologies are being explored which will allow smaller infusers to be developed and the first of these 'patch pumps' are already being marketed (see Chapter 9).

1.4 The pharmacology of CSII

Blood insulin profiles throughout the day during CSII more closely resemble those in the non-diabetic person than do standard insulin injection regimens, that is, there are clear peaks at mealtimes and a more constant basal level between meals and during the night. The improved control of CSII is most probably due to three main factors: the relatively flat basal blood insulin levels during CSII, particularly during the night, which cannot be achieved by long-acting insulin injections with their increase, peak, and decrease of insulin activity (Lepore *et al.* 2000); the ability to pre-programme a change in the basal rate which, for example, can counter a pre-breakfast blood glucose increase—the 'dawn phenomenon' (Koivisto *et al.* 1986); and the low variability of absorption of subcutaneously infused insulin (Lauritzen *et al.* 1983). The coefficient of variation for the absorption of isophane insulin is about ±50% and accounts for the marked day-to-day unpredictability in blood glucose levels in injection-treated type 1 diabetes. This can be reduced to below ±5% during CSII, thus reducing the within and between day variability of blood glucose concentrations (Chapter 2).

The steady-state plasma insulin levels achieved by either subcutaneous or intravenous insulin infusion at the same rate are similar, suggesting that there is little local subcutaneous insulin degradation during CSII. However, after a step increase in the basal rate, due to the delay in absorption of infused insulin, plasma insulin levels may take some hours to reach a new steady state (Kraegen and Chisholm 1985). This indicates that it is inadvisable to make too many basal rate changes in the CSII regimen—usually no more than about three are necessary.

1.5 Insulin pump therapy worldwide

CSII has gradually been incorporated into routine clinical practice for selected people with type 1 diabetes, encouraged by the availability of modern reliable pumps, greater clinical greater experience of pump therapy, the mounting evidence base for its effectiveness and the development of national guidelines outlining best practice, and the most appropriate clinical indications. Nevertheless, the uptake of CSII varies considerably around the world, from high-use countries such as the United States where about 35% (2009) of type 1 diabetic people use pump therapy to low-use countries such as the United Kingdom and Denmark (Figure 1.2). Surveys of physicians in countries where there is a low uptake of CSII indicate that the two main barriers to greater use are poor knowledge of the benefits and clinical indications for CSII by health care professionals and lack of resources to implement the treatment, exemplified by variable reimbursement of pumps and supplies by health services or insurance organizations and lack of trained staff to run insulin pump services (Nøgaard 2003). This leads to wide variations in the use of CSII even within countries.

Some of these problems are now being actively tackled by health services, manufacturers, diabetes associations, and others who are providing more education and training on insulin pump therapy, and by programmes to help local health organizations—both health care professionals and managers—implement clinical recommendations.

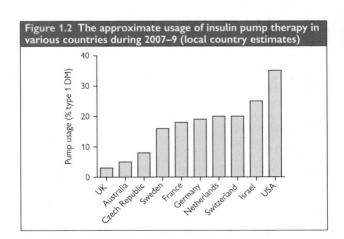

Figure 1.2 The approximate usage of insulin pump therapy in various countries during 2007–9 (local country estimates)

1.6 Guidelines and clinical indications for insulin pump therapy: NICE 2008

Several national guidelines for CSII have been formulated in recent years. A notable example is the report of the UK National Institute for Health and Clinical Excellence (NICE) which published a review and re-appraisal on CSII in 2008 (NICE 2008a). This was the result of a detailed examination of evidence submitted by many people and organizations including patients and patient groups, diabetes and other professional associations, manufacturers, clinical experts, local and central health departments, and research and guideline groups, as well as a comprehensive review on the clinical and cost-effectiveness of CSII commissioned by a Health Technology Assessment Group.

Although the NICE guidance concerns CSII use only in England and Wales, it is a good basis for the appropriate use of insulin pump therapy in most countries. Table 1.1 shows the 2008 NICE guidance for CSII.

The evidence base for the effectiveness of CSII is reviewed in Chapter 2 and this informs the clinical indications given in the Guidance. The rationales for the Guidance and some controversial points in the

---

Table 1.1 UK NICE guidance and clinical indications for CSII (2008)

CSII is recommended as a treatment option in type 1 diabetes:

(a) For adults and children 12 years of age and over when either:

Attempts to achieve target HbA$_{1c}$ levels with multiple daily insulin injections (MDI) result in disabling hypoglycaemia, or

HbA$_{1c}$ levels have remained high on MDI ($\geq$8.5%) despite a high level of care

(b) For children younger than 12 years when:

MDI is considered to be impractical or inappropriate, and with the expectation that children would be expected to undergo a later trial of MDI between the ages of 12 and 18 years.

Other notable points in the 2008 Guidance are as follows:

CSII should only be continued if there is sustained improvement in HbA$_{1c}$ or hypoglycaemia rate.

CSII should be initiated by a trained specialist team (see Chapter 3)—at least a diabetes physician with a special interest in insulin pump therapy, and a diabetes specialist nurse and dietitian trained in CSII.

When considering CSII in pregnant women with type 1 diabetes (see Chapter 6), the NICE guidance on Diabetes in Pregnancy (NICE 2008b) recommends CSII may be indicated when the target HbA$_{1c}$ of 6.1% or less pre-conceptually or in the first trimester cannot be achieved without the occurrence of disabling hypoglycaemia.

CSII is not generally recommended in type 2 diabetes though some subgroups may benefit (see Chapter 7) and more research is needed.

report have also been discussed recently (Pickup and Hammond 2009). Two points in particular are worth emphasizing. The choice by NICE of an $HbA_{1c} \geq 8.5\%$ as being the level of poor control at which CSII should be considered does not indicate the target HbA_{1c} that NICE recommends for type 1 diabetes management, but rather it is the level above which NICE judged CSII to be cost effective, *in the absence of disabling hypoglycaemia* (see Chapter 2 for a discussion of cost-effectiveness of insulin pump therapy). In fact, patients being considered for CSII because of continued unacceptable control during MDI, who have an HbA_{1c} below this level, are likely also to suffer from disabling hypoglycaemia and therefore warrant a trial of CSII under the guidance.

It will be noted that NICE recommends insulin pump therapy as an option in children with type 1 diabetes as well as for adults (see Chapter 5 for CSII in children and adolescents). In a change from earlier recommendations, NICE considers that children are no longer required to have 'failed on MDI' before being given a trial of CSII. Although we recommend that adult candidates for CSII should first have received best insulin injection therapy with MDI and renewed education, MDI is not always practical in some children, many being unable, unwilling, or prevented from injecting insulin at school, and sometimes restricted in activities because of the need to inject.

NICE has recommended that children started on CSII (who would therefore not yet have been treated by MDI in many cases) should subsequently undergo a trial of MDI between 12 and 18 years. But clinical and psychological problems may occur when changing the regimen in a teenager with well-controlled diabetes, particularly if MDI does not match the control of CSII. Whilst the option to stop CSII and trial MDI should be discussed with adolescents and parents, and will sometimes be a successful change, the physician may consider that the clinical, psychological, and social circumstances of an individual patient may sometimes indicate that a switch to MDI would not be advisable.

It should be noted that, apart from a reduction in hypoglycaemia and HbA_{1c}, several other benefits of CSII are recognized (Chapter 2), including improved blood glucose variability, better quality of life, and flexibility in lifestyle (particularly important in the shift worker, business person who travels extensively, and those with jobs where safety is essential). Although these are clearly important considerations for patients and are frequently mentioned as reasons for starting CSII (Bode *et al.* 2002), they have not yet been included in the NICE guidance. In some clinical practices, these indications are already acknowledged and we are likely to see more indications such as these added to national guidelines in the coming years.

References

Albisser AM, Leibel BS, Ewart TG *et al.* (1974). Clinical control of diabetes by the artificial pancreas. *Diabetes*, **23**, 397–404.

Bode BW, Tamborlane WV, and Davidson PC (2002). Insulin pump therapy in the 21st century. *Postgraduate Medicine*, **111**, 69–77.

Cahill GF, Etzweiler DD, and Freinkel N (1976). 'Control' and diabetes. *The New England Journal of Medicine*, **294**, 1004–5.

Champion MC, Shepherd GAA, Rodger NW, and Dupré J (1980). Continuous subcutaneous insulin infusion in the management of diabetes mellitus. *Diabetes*, **29**, 206–12.

Dahl-Jørgensen K, Brinchman-Hansen O, Hanssen KF *et al.* (1986). Effect of near-normoglycaemia for two years on the progression of early diabetic retinopathy: the Oslo Study. *British Medical Journal*, **293**, 1195–9.

Diabetes Control and Complications Trial Research Group (1993). The effect of intensive treatment of diabetes on the development and progression of long-term complications in insulin-dependent diabetes mellitus. *The New England Journal of Medicine*, **329**, 977–86.

Kadish AH (1963). Automation control of blood sugar. A servomechanism for glucose monitoring and control. *Transactions—American Society for Artificial Internal Organs*, **19**, 363–7.

Koivisto VA, Yki-Järvinen H, Helve E, and Pelkonen R (1986). Pathogenesis and prevention of the dawn phenomenon in diabetic patients treated with CSII. *Diabetes*, **35**, 78–82.

Kraegen EW and Chisholm DJ (1985). Pharmacokinetics of insulin. Implications for continuous subcutaneous insulin infusion therapy. *Clinical Pharmacokinetics*, **10**, 303–14.

Kroc Collaborative Study Group (1984). Blood glucose control and the evolution of diabetic retinopathy and albuminuria. *The New England Journal of Medicine*, **311**, 365–72.

Lauritzen T, Pramming S, Deckert T, and Binder C (1983). Pharmacokinetics of continuous subcutaneous insulin infusion. *Diabetologia*, **24**, 326–9.

Lepore M, Pampanelli S, Fanelli C *et al.* (2000). Pharmacokinetics and pharmacodynamics of subcutaneous injection of long-acting human insulin analog glargine, NPH insulin, and ultralente human insulin and continuous subcutaneous infusion of insulin lispro. *Diabetes*, **49**, 2142–8.

Mecklenburg RS, Benson JW, Becker NM *et al.* (1982). Clinical use of the insulin infusion pump in 100 patients with type 1 diabetes. *The New England Journal of Medicine*, **307**, 513–18.

NICE (National Institute for Health and Clinical Excellence) (2008a). Continuous subcutaneous insulin infusion for the treatment of diabetes mellitus. Technology Appraisal Guidance 151 (Review of Technology Appraisal Guidance 57). NICE, London.

NICE (National Institute for Health and Clinical Excellence) (2008b). Diabetes in pregnancy. Clinical Guideline 63. NICE, London.

Nøgaard K (2003). A nationwide study of continuous subcutaneous insulin infusion (CSII) in Denmark. *Diabetic Medicine*, **20**, 307–11.

Pfeiffer EF, Thum CH, and Clemens AH (1974). The artificial beta-cell. A continuous control of blood sugar by external regulation of insulin infusion (glucose-controlled insulin infusion system). *Hormone and Metabolic Research*, **6**, 339–42.

Pickup JC and Hammond P (2009). NICE guidance on continuous subcutaneous insulin infusion 2008: review of the Technology Appraisal Guidance. *Diabetic Medicine*, **26**, 1–4.

Pickup JC, Keen H, Parsons JA, and Alberti KGMM (1978). Continuous subcutaneous insulin infusion: an approach to achieving normoglycaemia. *British Medical Journal*, I, 204–7.

Pickup JC, Keen H, Parsons JA, Alberti KGMM, and Rowe AS (1979a). Continuous subcutaneous insulin infusion: improved blood glucose and intermediary metabolite control in diabetes. *Lancet*, i, 1255–8.

Pickup JC, White MC, Keen H, Kohner EM, Parsons JA, and Alberti KGMM (1979b). Long-term continuous subcutaneous insulin infusion in diabetics at home. *Lancet*, ii, 870–3.

Slama G, Hautecouvature M, Assan R, and Tchobroutsky G (1974). One to five days of continuous insulin infusion on seven diabetic patients. *Diabetes*, **23**, 732–8.

Steno Study Group (1982). Effect of 6 months of strict metabolic control on eye and kidney function in insulin-dependent diabetics with background retinopathy. *Lancet*, i, 121–4.

Tamborlane WV, Sherwin RS, Genel M, and Felig P (1979a). Reduction to normal of plasma glucose in juvenile diabetes by subcutaneous administration of insulin with a portable infusion pump. *The New England Journal of Medicine*, **300**, 573–8.

Tamborlane WV, Sherwin RS, Genel M, and Felig P (1979b). Restoration of normal lipid and amino acid metabolism in diabetic patients treated with a portable insulin-infusion pump. *Lancet*, i, 1258–61.

Chapter 2

The evidence base for insulin pump therapy

John Pickup

Key points

- All grades of hypoglycaemia are less during continuous subcutaneous insulin infusion (CSII) than during multiple daily insulin injections (MDI) treatment. The mean frequency of severe hypoglycaemia is about 75% less on CSII vs. MDI, with the greatest reduction occurring in those with most hypoglycaemia on MDI
- Meta-analysis of randomized controlled trials (RCTs) and before/after studies shows that the mean difference in HbA$_{1c}$ between MDI and CSII is about 0.5%–0.6%, but the worst controlled subjects on MDI enjoy the greatest improvement on switching to CSII. Those with an HbA$_{1c}$ of 9%–10% on MDI may see a reduction of 3%–4% on CSII. Glycaemic variability is also improved on switching to CSII
- Other benefits of CSII include a reduction in the dawn phenomenon, reduced daily insulin dosage, and improved quality of life
- Health economic studies indicate that CSII is a cost-effective use of resources

There is now good evidence that in many people with type 1 diabetes insulin pump therapy provides significant advantages compared to best insulin injection therapy, usually considered to be multiple daily insulin injections (MDI) (Box 2.1). In particular, the frequency of all grades of hypoglycaemia is reduced and there is improved glycaemic control as measured by HbA$_{1c}$. In addition, the benefits of continuous subcutaneous insulin infusion (CSII) include reduced glycaemic variability, reduced insulin dosage, and improved quality of life and well-being. Nevertheless, CSII is more expensive than insulin injection treatment and since all health care systems in the world are cash-limited, the

Box 2.1 The benefits of insulin pump

Reduction in
- Severe, moderate, and mild hypoglycaemia
- Mean blood glucose concentration and HbA_{1c}
- Within- and between-day blood glucose variability
- Daily insulin dosage
- Risk of microvascular disease

Improvement in
- Patient's satisfaction with therapy
- Quality of life and well-being

cost-effectiveness must be carefully considered. In this chapter, the clinical and health economic evidence basis for the use of CSII in type 1 diabetes in routine clinical practice is summarized. The possible benefits of insulin pump therapy in type 2 diabetes are discussed in Chapter 7.

2.1 Hypoglycaemia reduction

Hypoglycaemia is a major problem in type 1 diabetes and is widely thought to be the greatest barrier to improving control. This is illustrated by the observation that since the publication of the Diabetes Control and Complications Trial (DCCT) in 1993 there have been strenuous efforts made to improve control in diabetes but, frustratingly, as HbA_{1c} has been lowered year after year, the frequency of severe hypoglycaemia (where third party assistance is needed) has increased (Bulsara et al. 2004).

Several early studies in the 1980s indicated that the frequency of severe hypoglycaemia during insulin pump therapy was less than during either conventional insulin injection therapy (CIT) or the intensified regimen of MDI. For example, we found that the rate of severe hypoglycaemia in a group of 40 patients with type 1 diabetes treated by CSII for >6 months was about one-third of that in a matched group of type 1 subjects managed by CIT (Bending et al. 1985b). Also, in a randomized controlled trial (RCT) of CSII vs. either MDI or CIT (the 'Oslo Study'), the frequency of severe hypoglycaemia was reduced from 14 episodes on MDI to two episodes on pump therapy (p < 0.001) (Dahl-Jørgensen et al. 1986).

Further studies in the 1990s underlined the potential of CSII to reduce hypoglycaemia. In an observational trial of insulin pump therapy over 4 years, Bode et al. (1996) recorded an approximately 78% reduction in severe hypoglycaemia when patients with type 1 diabetes were switched from MDI to CSII, even though HbA_{1c} levels were comparable during the two therapies (7.7% vs. 7.4%, MDI vs. CSII). In another study in adolescents who chose either CSII or MDI treatment, HbA_{1c} was lower in the pump group after 6 months treatment (7.7% vs. 8.1%, p = 0.003, CSII vs. MDI), but nonetheless the frequency of severe hypoglycaemia was reduced by nearly 50% in those managed by CSII (Boland et al. 1999).

In a recent meta-analysis of the efficacy of the modern practice of CSII (Pickup and Sutton 2008), we specifically compared the frequency of severe hypoglycaemia during MDI and CSII, considering only trials published after 1996 (i.e. using modern pumps and monomeric insulins), where the duration of pump therapy was ≥6 months (i.e. long enough for severe hypoglycaemia to be accurately assessed) and in patients with a significant initial hypoglycaemia rate on MDI (≥10 episodes/100 patient-years). In 22 studies in 21 trials, the rate ratio (RR) for severe hypoglycaemia was reduced by about 75% on switching to CSII (mean RR 4.19 [95% confidence interval 2.86–6.13]), with no significant difference between the RR in RCTs and observational before/after studies (Figure 2.1). The greatest effect in reducing hypoglycaemia by CSII occurred in those with the highest rates during MDI. Meta-regression also indicated that pump therapy reduces severe hypoglycaemia in both adults and children, though the RR for hypoglycaemia reduction is slightly lower in children. This is probably explained by the lower diabetes duration and therefore the lower frequency of hypoglycaemia during MDI in children (in this meta-analysis, a mean hypoglycaemia rate of 36 vs. 100 episodes/100 patient-years, children vs. adults).

Lesser degrees of mild or moderate hypoglycaemia are also a frequent occurrence in MDI-treated type 1 diabetes, and are significantly reduced by pump therapy. We found that the percentage of self-monitored blood glucose values <3.5mmol/L (63mg/dL) was reduced from about 10% to 2.5% (p = 0.03) by changing from MDI to CSII (Pickup et al. 2005).

2.2 **Improvement in glycaemic control and HbA$_{1c}$**

Comparisons of glycaemic control during MDI and CSII have been somewhat confusing over the years. An initial meta-analysis of 12 RCTs comparing MDI and CSII indicated that the mean difference in HbA_{1c} and mean blood glucose concentration between the two treatments, though significantly favouring CSII, was relatively unimpressive at about 0.5% and 1mmol/L (18mg/dL), respectively (Pickup et al. 2002). However, our more recent meta-analysis mentioned

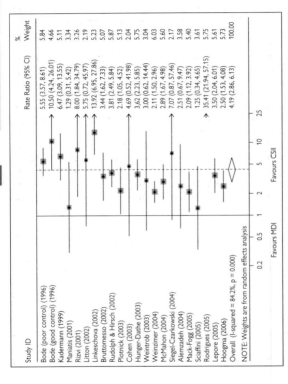

Figure 2.1 Meta-analysis of 22 studies comparing the rate ratio for severe hypoglycaemia during MDI vs. severe hypoglycaemia is reduced by a mean of 4.19-fold on switching from MDI to CSII. Data from Pickup and Sutton (2008); see original reference for details of studies.

Study ID	Rate Ratio (95% CI)	% Weight
Bode (poor control) (1996)	5.55 (3.57, 8.61)	5.84
Bode (good control) (1996)	10.50 (4.24, 26.01)	4.66
Kadermann (1999)	6.47 (3.09, 13.55)	5.11
Maniatis (2001)	1.29 (0.31, 5.42)	3.34
Rizvi (2001)	8.00 (1.84, 34.79)	3.26
Litton (2002)	5.75 (0.72, 45.97)	2.19
Linkeschova (2002)	13.92 (6.95, 27.86)	5.23
Bruttomesso (2002)	3.44 (1.62, 7.33)	5.07
Rudolph & Hirsch (2002)	3.81 (2.49, 5.84)	5.87
Plotnick (2003)	2.18 (1.05, 4.52)	5.13
Cohen (2003)	4.69 (0.52, 41.98)	2.04
Hunger-Dathe (2003)	3.62 (2.23, 5.85)	5.75
Weintrob (2003)	3.00 (0.62, 14.44)	3.04
Weinzimer (2004)	2.11 (1.50, 2.96)	6.03
McMahon (2004)	2.89 (1.67, 4.98)	5.60
Siegel-Czarkowski (2004)	7.07 (0.87, 57.46)	2.17
Alemzadeh (2004)	2.51 (0.67, 9.47)	3.58
Mack-Fogg (2005)	2.09 (1.12, 3.92)	5.40
Sciaffini (2005)	1.25 (0.34, 4.65)	3.61
Rodrigues (2005)	35.41 (21.94, 57.15)	5.75
Lepore (2005)	3.50 (2.04, 6.01)	5.61
Hoogma (2006)	2.50 (1.53, 4.08)	5.73
Overall (I-squared = 84.2%, p = 0.000)	4.19 (2.86, 6.13)	100.00

NOTE: Weights are from random effects analysis

Favours MDI   Favours CSII

earlier (Pickup and Sutton 2008) has shown that, as with hypoglycaemia reduction, the greatest glycaemic improvement occurs in the worst controlled patients on MDI. For example, in trials with a mean HbA$_{1c}$ of ~9.5% on MDI, the reduction in mean HbA$_{1c}$ on transferring to CSII was about 1.5%. This notion that CSII is most effective in poorly controlled patients has also been confirmed in individual subjects, both in a pooled analysis of those who took part in three RCTs (Retnakaran et al. 2004) and in audits of patients in insulin pump clinics (Pickup et al. 2006). Individual patients with an HbA$_{1c}$ of 10%–12% on MDI can drop their HbA$_{1c}$ by 3%–4% during insulin pump therapy (Figure 2.2).

It is important to note that many people with type 1 diabetes who are referred to insulin pump clinics will have a high HbA$_{1c}$, in spite of best attempts to control their diabetes over many years with MDI, and in spite of reporting significant hypoglycaemia (Pickup et al. 2005). In our recent meta-analysis (Pickup and Sutton 2008), the mean HbA$_{1c}$ on MDI was >8.5% in 10 trials (mean 9.0%), even in the face of severe hypoglycaemia at a mean rate of 65 episodes/100 patient-years. Since a major determinant of the level of HbA$_{1c}$ that can be achieved on MDI is the degree of glycaemic variability (Pickup et al. 2006), one may speculate that hypoglycaemia-prone patients with wide swings in blood glucose choose to maintain an elevated HbA$_{1c}$ to avoid precipitating unpleasant hypoglycaemia as attempts are made to tighten control on MDI.

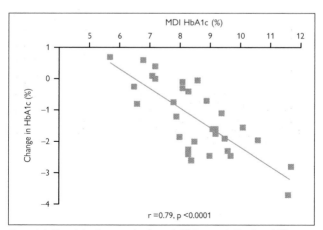

Figure 2.2 Correlation between the change in HbA$_{1c}$ on switching from MDI to CSII and the initial HbA$_{1c}$ during MDI in subjects with type 1 diabetes. The greatest effect of CSII at lowering HbA$_{1c}$ is in the worst controlled patients. From Pickup et al. (2006).

2.3 **Reduction in blood glucose variability**

Wide variations in blood glucose levels both within and between days is a characteristic of and a frustration for many people with type 1 diabetes. Unpredictable swings in blood glucose are possibly a more common presenting complaint to some Insulin Pump Clinics than hypoglycaemia. CSII reduces both types of variation: the within-day variability of self-monitored blood glucose values (measured as the interquartile range of daily tests), is reduced by about 40%, and the day-to-day variability (measured by the interquartile range of successive fasting blood glucose tests) by about 50% on switching to pump therapy (Pickup *et al.* 2006). Many studies have noted improvement in within-day variability during CSII, though the day-to-day predictability of glycaemia on MDI and CSII has been less well researched.

The most important factor leading to unpredictable control in type 1 diabetes treated by insulin injection therapy is probably the large variation in the subcutaneous absorption of long-acting insulin formulations. CSII reduces the variation in insulin absorption from about ±50% with isophane insulin to about ±3% on pump therapy (Lauritzen *et al.* 1983). This is probably because of the very small subcutaneous depot of insulin at any one time during CSII (~1 unit) and the reduced effects that variations in subcutaneous blood flow have on small insulin doses.

2.4 **The impact of long-acting insulin analogues**

The newer long-acting insulin analogues, glargine and detemir, have flatter insulin profiles and more predictable absorption than isophane or lente insulins and have improved glycaemic control in many people with type 1 diabetes. It is reasonable to ask if they have removed the need for insulin pump therapy.

Evidence to date indicates that a lower HbA_{1c} can be achieved by CSII than analogue-based MDI. We have found that in those patients referred to our Insulin Pump Clinic who were initially receiving isophane-MDI, the HbA_{1c} remained at a similar level when they were transferred to glargine-MDI in an attempt to improve control in the pre-pump assessment programme (see Chapter 3) (Pickup and Renard 2008). Subsequent switching to CSII resulted in a significant fall in HbA_{1c} from 8.7 ± 1.2% to 7.2 ± 1.0% (mean ± SD, p <0.001; see Figure 2.3). In a meta-analysis of 4 trials comparing HbA_{1c} during glargine-MDI vs. CSII, the mean difference of 0.63% was similar to the mean difference of 0.62% between isophane-MDI and CSII (Pickup and Sutton 2008). Finally, an RCT in type 1 diabetic subjects allocated to either glargine/aspart-MDI or CSII with aspart insulin showed that a significantly lower HbA_{1c} was achieved with CSII (Doyle *et al.* 2004).

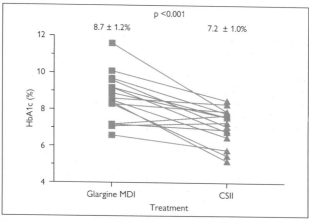

Figure 2.3 HbA1c levels in subjects with type 1 diabetes treated by glargine-based MDI and then subsequently switched to CSII. From Pickup and Renard (2008).

There have been no long-term, adequately sized head-to-head RCTs comparing severe hypoglycaemia during glargine- or detemir-MDI vs. CSII. However, the frequency of severe hypoglycaemia is not usually reduced by glargine or detemir vs. isophane-MDI (Home *et al.* 2004; Warren *et al.* 2004). With the earlier evidence then, and when insulin pump clinics operate a sequential strategy where no patient is offered a trial of CSII unless their clinical problems of hypoglycaemia and/or elevated HbA_{1c} remain on optimized MDI, with long-acting analogues if necessary (Chapter 3), it is reasonable to conclude that glargine and detemir have not replaced the need for insulin pump therapy.

2.5 Reduction in the dawn phenomenon

The 'dawn phenomenon' is an increase in the blood glucose concentration in the few hours before breakfast, and is a common problem in insulin injection-treated type 1 diabetes. It is due to a combination of waning of blood insulin levels from the previous evening's delayed-action insulin injection and increasing insulin resistance caused by nocturnal growth hormone surges. With the introduction of long-acting insulin analogues such as glargine and detemir, this dawn blood glucose increase is less common but is still a significant cause of clinical problems. Patients typically complain that attempts to lower the fasting blood glucose level by increasing the evening long-acting insulin result in nocturnal hypoglycaemia.

CSII has a major advantage over injection therapy in that the basal rate can be preset to increase at some point during the night and thus counter the dawn phenomenon (Koivisto et al. 1986). Even when using a single basal rate throughout the 24 hours, the dawn phenomenon is quite rare during CSII (Bending et al. 1985a), presumably because the more constant nocturnal blood insulin levels avoid the element of the pre-breakfast hyperglycaemia due to evening long-acting insulin 'running out'.

2.6 **Reduction in insulin dose**

It is well established that the improved glycaemic control which is seen during CSII is achieved at a lower daily insulin dose than that used on MDI. We found in a meta-analysis of 12 RCTs comparing MDI and CSII that the mean insulin dose was reduced by about 14% (Pickup et al. 2002) and in an audit of our insulin pump clinic 28% less insulin was used in the pump patients when switched from MDI (Pickup et al. 2005). This is the basis for the common strategy when starting insulin pump patients of using a total daily dose which is 20% of the previous dose on injections (see Chapter 3).

Apart from the cost savings, a reduced insulin dosage on CSII contributes to the lowered risk of hypoglycaemia and helps with weight control.

2.7 **Reduced risk of microvascular disease**

The relationship between HbA_{1c} and microvascular risk as defined by the DCCT is curvilinear (i.e. steeper at higher HbA_{1c} levels). As previously mentioned, many patients who are candidates for CSII have an elevated HbA_{1c} at referral on injection therapy, and this is a recognized indication for a trial of CSII in many national guidelines (Chapter 1) (NICE 2008). Reducing the HbA_{1c} from, say, 10% on MDI to just 8% on CSII (which would be predicted from Figure 2.2) will reduce the risk of developing sustained retinopathy progression, for example, by about 4 cases per 100 patient-years. In other words, treatment by CSII for 10 years would reduce the number of patients developing retinopathy in this poor-control group by about 40%. This is much higher than the original estimates of about a 5% risk reduction for microvascular disease in the general type 1 diabetic subjects when improved by a mean HbA_{1c} of 0.5% on pump therapy (Pickup et al. 2002).

2.8 Improved treatment satisfaction and quality of life

Formal measures comparing quality of life (QoL) during MDI and CSII have given variable results, with some studies indicating no significant difference between injection- and pump-treated subjects (Tsui *et al.* 2001), but more studies showing a significant improvement on pump therapy (DeVries *et al.* 2002; Linkeschova *et al.* 2002; McMahon *et al.* 2005; Pickup and Harris 2007).

This discrepancy may be because measuring QoL is notoriously difficult. Most popular indices like the Diabetes Quality of Life score developed by the DCCT ask questions about predetermined domains which the health care professional considers important for QoL—pain, mood, insulin injections, complications, and so on. Whereas, the patient might rate a happy family life, the ability to enjoy a hobby, or sound personal finances more important than feeling well. Patient-centred measures of QoL, where the person with diabetes nominates and grades what he or she considers important, rate QoL better on CSII than MDI (Pickup and Harris 2007).

Examples of RCTs which have compared QoL during MDI and CSII include that of DeVries *et al.* (2002) where in 79 type 1 diabetic subjects allocated to MDI or CSII over 16 weeks, the general health score was significantly better on pump therapy. Several observational studies support an improved QoL during CSII (Linkeschova *et al.* 2002; McMahon *et al.* 2005; Pickup and Harris 2007).

2.9 Cost-effectiveness

Several studies have compared the cost-effectiveness of MDI and CSII, and most of the modelling has found CSII to be cost effective (Roze *et al.* 2005; Cohen *et al.* 2007). The treatment costs of insulin pump therapy include the capital cost of the pump, which in the United Kingdom is about £2,400 to £2,750, with a 4–6 year warranty. Although the lifetime for the pump maybe some 7 years, as new and improved pump models are introduced they are generally not used much beyond the warranty period, giving an annualized cost of about £500–600. The consumable costs of pump therapy relate to infusion sets and reservoirs (about £1,200 per annum), in addition to the blood glucose monitoring and insulin (albeit with less insulin) costs common to MDI, with a total consumables cost of about £2,000 per annum. The additional costs of training (staff and patients), and medical, nursing, and dietitian time which is over and above that incurred in MDI is not well defined, will vary from one centre to another according to experience and procedures and is sometimes not included in cost-effectiveness estimates.

Assuming insulin, needle, and pen costs for MDI of about £900 per annum (with the same blood testing as CSII), the annualized cost of pump therapy at about £2,500 is some £1,600 greater than MDI.

The cost-effectiveness of pump therapy is modelled from the expected reduction in mean blood glucose concentration and HbA_{1c} and thus the reduced risk of diabetes complications and the reduction in hypoglycaemia. Hypoglycaemia is a major influence on the QoL of patients and the satisfaction they have with their treatment, a main determinant of the quality of control that can be achieved and one of the greatest fears of people with diabetes, but the financial cost of hypoglycaemia is not always huge. Many episodes of even severe hypoglycaemia do not result in an emergency room visit or hospital admission and thus one of the major benefits of CSII has a low impact on cost-effectiveness calculations.

Most estimates of cost-effectiveness are dependent on the baseline HbA_{1c}, on MDI (since CSII is most effective in the worst controlled patients; Figure 2.2), with an ICER (incremental cost-effectiveness ratio) varying from about £17,000 to £35,000 per quality adjusted life year (QALY) gained, depending on the report, the assumed HbA_{1c} level on MDI, and the expected reduction on switching to CSII.

In a recent review of CSII and guidance on its use (NICE 2008), the UK National Institute for Health and Clinical Excellence considered that, *based on HbA_{1c} alone*, pump treatment was not cost effective at HbA_{1c} levels on MDI below about 9% unless QoL improvements, which are not captured in the usual models, are included. (Since it is known that QoL does improve on CSII, NICE therefore judged it to be cost effective when HbA_{1c} levels on MDI are ≥8.5%.) NICE considered that avoiding hypoglycaemia and the associated reduced fear of this complication might result in an increase in QoL—a 0.01 increase would decrease the ICER to £29,300 and a 0.03 increase in QoL change the ICER to £21,000 per QALY gained. NICE has a threshold range for acceptable cost-effectiveness of £20,000–£30,000 per QALY gained.

These calculations therefore show that that CSII is a clear cost-effective use of resources for the two main clinical indications of elevated HbA_{1c} and disabling hypoglycaemia during MDI.

References

Bending JJ, Pickup JC, Collins ACG, and Keen H (1985a). Rarity of a marked 'dawn phenomenon' in diabetic subjects treated by continuous subcutaneous insulin infusion. *Diabetes Care*, **8**, 28–33.

Bending JJ, Pickup JC, and Keen H (1985b). Frequency of diabetic ketoacidosis and hypoglycemic coma during treatment with continuous subcutaneous insulin infusion: an audit of medical care. *The American Journal of Medicine*, **79**, 685–91.

Bode BW, Steed RD, and Davidson PC (1996). Reduction in severe hypoglycemia with long-term continuous subcutaneous insulin infusion in type 1 diabetes. *Diabetes Care*, **19**, 324–7.

Boland EA, Grey M, Oesterle A, Fredrickson L, and Tamborlane WV (1999). Continuous subcutaneous insulin infusion. A new way to lower risk of severe hypoglycemia, improve metabolic control and enhance coping in adolescents with type 1 diabetes. *Diabetes Care*, **22**, 1799–84.

Bulsara MK, Holman CDJ, Davis EA, and Jones TW (2004). The impact of a decade of changing treatment on rates of severe hypoglycemia in a population-based cohort of children with type 1 diabetes. *Diabetes Care*, **27**, 2293–8.

Cohen N, Minshall ME, Sharon-Nash L, Zakrzewska K, Valentine WJ, and Palmer AJ (2007). Continuous subcutaneous insulin infusion versus multiple daily injections of insulin in adult and adolescent type 1 diabetes mellitus in Australia. *Phamacoeconomics*, **25**, 881–97.

Dahl-Jørgensen K, Brinchman-Hansen O, Hanssen KF *et al.* (1986). Effect of near-normoglycaemia for two years on the progression of early diabetic retinopathy: the Oslo Study. *British Medical Journal*, **293**, 1195–9.

DeVries JH, Snoek FJ, Kostense PJ *et al.* (2002). A randomized trial of continuous subcutaneous insulin infusion and intensive injection therapy in type 1 diabetes for patients with long-standing poor glycemic control. *Diabetes Care*, **25**, 2074–80.

Doyle EA, Weinzimer SA, Steffen AT, Ahern JA, Vincent M, and Tamborlane WV (2004). A randomized, prospective trial comparing the efficacy of continuous subcutaneous insulin infusion with multiple daily injections using insulin glargine. *Diabetes Care*, **27**, 1554–8.

Home P, Bartley P, Russell-Jones D *et al.* (2004). Insulin detemir offers improved glycemic control compared to NPH insulin in people with type 1 diabetes. *Diabetes Care*, **27**, 1081–7.

Koivisto VA, Yki-Järvinen H, Helve E, and Pelkonen R (1986). Pathogenesis and prevention of the dawn phenomenon in diabetic patients treated with CSII. *Diabetes*, **35**, 78–82.

Lauritzen T, Pramming S, Deckert T, and Binder C (1983). Pharmacokinetics of continuous subcutaneous insulin infusion. *Diabetologia*, **24**, 326–9.

Linkeschova R, Raoul M, Bott U, Berger M, and Spraul M (2002). Less severe hypoglycaemia, better metabolic control, and improved quality of life in type 1 diabetes mellitus with continuous subcutaneous insulin infusion (CSII) therapy; an observational study of 100 consecutive patients followed for a mean of 2 years. *Diabetic Medicine*, **219**, 746–751.

McMahon SK, Airey FL, Marangou DA *et al.* (2005). Insulin pump therapy in children and adolescents: improvements in key parameters of diabetes management including quality of life. *Diabetic Medicine*, **22**, 92–96.

NICE (National Institute for Health and Clinical Excellence) (2008). Continuous subcutaneous insulin infusion for the treatment of diabetes mellitus. Technology Appraisal Guidance 151 (Review of Technology Appraisal Guidance 57). NICE, London.

Pickup JC and Harris A (2007). Assessing quality of life for new diabetes treatments and technologies: a simple patient-centered score. *Journal of Diabetes Science and Technology*, **1**, 394–9.

Pickup JC and Renard E (2008). Long-acting insulin analogues versus insulin pump therapy for the treatment of type 1 and type 2 diabetes. *Diabetes Care*, **31**, S140–5.

Pickup JC and Sutton AJ (2008). Severe hypoglycaemia and glycaemic control in type 1 diabetes: meta-analysis of multiple daily insulin injections versus continuous subcutaneous insulin infusion. *Diabetic Medicine*, **25**, 765–74.

Pickup JC, Mattock MB, and Kerry S (2002). Glycaemic control with continuous subcutaneous insulin infusion compared to intensive insulin injection therapy in type 1 diabetes: meta-analysis of randomised controlled trials. *British Medical Journal*, **324**, 705–8.

Pickup JC, Kidd J, Burmiston S, and Yemane N (2005). Effectiveness of continuous subcutaneous insulin infusion in hypoglycaemia-prone type 1 diabetes: implications for NICE guidelines. *Practical Diabetes International*, **22**, 10–14.

Pickup JC, Kidd J, Burmiston S, and Yemane N (2006). Determinants of glycaemic control in type 1 diabetes during intensified therapy with multiple daily insulin injections or continuous subcutaneous insulin infusion: importance of blood glucose variability. *Diabetes/Metabolism Research and Reviews*, **22**, 232–7.

Retnakaran R, Hochman J, DeVries JH et al. (2004). Continuous subcutaneous insulin infusion versus multiple daily injections. The impact of baseline A1c. *Diabetes Care*, **27**, 2590–6.

Roze S, Valentine WJ, Zakrzewska KE, and Palmer AJ (2005). Health-economic comparison of continuous subcutaneous insulin infusion with multiple daily injection for the treatment of type 1 diabetes in the UK. *Diabetic Medicine*, **22**, 1239–45.

Tsui E, Barnie A, Ross S, Parkes R, and Zinman B (2001). Intensive insulin therapy with insulin lispro. A randomised trial of continuous subcutaneous insulin infusion versus multiple daily injection. *Diabetes Care*, **24**, 1722–7.

Warren E, Weatherley-Jones E, Chilcott J, and Beverley C (2004). Systematic review and economic evaluation of a long-acting insulin analogue, insulin glargine. *Health Technology Assessment*, **8**(45), 1–57.

Chapter 3

Running an insulin pump service

John Pickup, Siobhan Pender, Julia Kidd, Nardos Yemane

Key points

- Patients are selected for continuous subcutaneous insulin infusion (CSII) because they meet clinical criteria (e.g. disabling hypoglycaemia and/or elevated HbA$_{1c}$ on multiple daily insulin injections [MDI]), general requirements (e.g. willing and able to perform pump procedures), and have no obvious contraindications, for example, unwilling or unable to perform pump procedures

- A sequential approach to treatment by CSII is recommended where patients first undergo a pre-pump assessment (including renewed diabetes education, optimization on MDI, for at least adults), with only those not achieving good control being offered a trial of pump therapy

- Basal insulin rates are about 50% of the total daily dose and meal boluses are set by the insulin: carbohydrate ratio and a correction factor based on the insulin sensitivity factor for the individual

- Dietitians play a crucial role in the pump service in teaching carbohydrate counting, preventing weight gain, treating and avoiding hypoglycaemia, and promoting healthy eating

- CSII is typically started as an outpatient; education and training are vital

3.1 Patient selection

People with diabetes are normally selected for a trial of insulin pump therapy if they meet three requirements: (1) the specific clinical indications for treatment by continuous subcutaneous insulin infusion (CSII) stipulated by the country's health service (e.g. NICE Guidance in the United Kingdom) or the insurance organization that is reimbursing the cost of CSII; (2) the general requirements in patients for best results from pump therapy; and (3) the absence of relative contraindications for CSII (see Box 3.1). The health care team supervising insulin pump therapy in those patients who are self-funding and not seeking approval and reimbursement from health organizations may also consider these selection requirements for best practice.

3.1.1 Clinical indications

The clinical indications for insulin pump therapy used in the United Kingdom and given by NICE (NICE 2008a) are outlined in Chapter 1 and in brief they are adults with type 1 diabetes who have disabling hypoglycaemia or an elevated HbA_{1c} ($\geq 8.5\%$), in spite of a high level of care with multiple dose insulin injections (MDI). These indications are similar to those of several health care organizations throughout the world. NICE also recommends CSII as a treatment option in children under 12 years of age who (like adults) have failed to achieve an acceptable HbA_{1c} or who have experienced disabling hypoglycaemia but (unlike in adults) this may be considered without a trial of MDI, if this is judged clinically inappropriate or impractical. This is because many paediatric diabetologists and parents consider that multiple, small insulin doses in very young children and midday insulin injections at school make MDI impractical in many children and render strict control difficult to achieve on this regimen (Pickup and Hammond 2009; see Chapter 5).

Several additional benefits of CSII are described in Chapter 2 and, of these, improved quality of life and well-being are notable and impressively articulated by patients in surveys and in the Insulin Pump Clinic. Aspects of pump therapy that impinge upon quality of life include the lifestyle flexibility afforded by the ability to delay or omit meals, the ease of adjusting basal insulin to counter exercise-induced hypoglycaemia or stress-induced hyperglycaemia, the increase in energy, the disappearance of irritability and tiredness, and the renewed confidence to face a demanding working day without hypoglycaemia. These important benefits have not yet been incorporated as reasons for trialling CSII in many national guidelines (e.g. NICE), though suboptimal quality of life on MDI may well be added to some criteria in the near future. Equally, CSII is generally not recommended as a treatment option for type 2 diabetes (NICE 2008a), though several case reports of people with uncontrolled, often insulin-resistant type 2 diabetes on MDI who improve markedly after a switch to CSII (Nielsen et al. 2005) argues that individual cases should be considered by the health care team (see Chapter 7).

3.1.2 General requirements (Box 3.1)

It goes without saying that patients must be willing to undertake insulin pump therapy (after discussion and explanation of CSIII—see later) and not to have this forced upon them by the health care team. Moreover, CSII works best in those who have certain positive key attitudes to their diabetes:

- *Acceptance of diabetes.* It is helpful for the patient to be comfortable and confident discussing diabetes (and ultimately the insulin pump) with friends, family, and colleagues. Those who do not accept many aspects of diabetes, say the need for frequent insulin injections and blood glucose monitoring, tend to not accept the pump. But health care professionals should be aware that there are demotivated, frustrated patients who cannot get good control on insulin injections and who thus do not readily 'accept' their diabetes, but who can sometimes use the tool of insulin pump therapy to improve control and to be rewarded and motivated by its effectiveness (see motivation).

- *Acceptance and trust of technology, rules, and protocols.* Although it is true that the young more readily accept technology, CSII has been successfully used by those of all age groups, social classes, and levels of educational ability. Some may take longer to come to terms with the technology than others, and pump procedures include adherence to protocols as well as just 'pressing the pump buttons'.

- *Motivation.* It is frequently said that pump patients must be highly motivated. Whilst this is true for the best results, in our experience and, as expected, people who have had poor control of diabetes and a poor quality of life for many years, who have serious complications or know they are at major risk, are usually motivated to do anything that will improve their lot. Indeed, sometimes they have erroneously been told that their frequent hypoglycaemia or elevated HbA_{1c} is because they have not been motivated enough with their diabetes treatment to date.

- *Having realistic expectations.* This requirement has some of the pitfalls of 'motivation', and is often mentioned. It should be explained that pump therapy is not a cure, not an artificial pancreas, and not an easy option which requires little patient input, but few think it is. On the contrary, many pump candidates are desperate and depressed after years of poor control and have limited expectations that something can improve their control.

- *Ability and willingness to master the procedures of CSII.* Though it is often said that those with poor cognition, vision, or dexterity may struggle with pump therapy, we have found that there are few who fall into this category, particularly if the simpler pump regimens are used for certain individuals (without bolus calculators, different meal profiles, etc). Key procedures which must be learnt include carbohydrate counting and adjustment of insulin dosages at meals, and frequent blood glucose monitoring, at least 4–6 times daily.

3.1.3 **Relative contraindications (Box 3.1)**

CSII will not be successful without a team of health care professionals (physician, nurse, and dietitian) trained and competent in this therapy, and their absence is an absolute contraindication. Major psychiatric illness is a contraindication. Patients with certain types of 'brittle diabetes' have historically performed poorly on CSII (Pickup *et al.* 1983). This applies particularly to the group of young, often female, apparently insulin-resistant type 1 diabetic people who have had multiple admissions to hospital with ketoacidosis. Often deliberate self-interference with treatment has been suspected in this group (Schade *et al.* 1985), and CSII presents several opportunities for malefaction (which we have seen), including dilution of the insulin, reversal of batteries, and removal of the delivery cannulae. Conversely, there are several case reports of patients with ketoacidosis-prone brittle diabetes who have been seen reduced episodes of ketoacidosis and admissions with CSII (Blackett 1995), though usually not with near-normalization of metabolic control. Probably, maintaining enough insulin to avoid most ketosis with the basal delivery but without reliance on compliance, and more positive interactions with staff are important factors in any success. However, brittle diabetes should be treated cautiously by CSII.

Box 3.1 Patient selection for insulin pump therapy

Clinical indications for a trial of CSII:

- Disabling hypoglycaemia in type 1 diabetes during MDI (adults)
- Elevated HbA$_{1c}$ in type 1 diabetes during MDI (adults)
- Hypoglycaemia or elevated HbA$_{1c}$ in children with type 1 diabetes but without the need for MDI
- Other indications as agreed by the national health service or funder (e.g. suboptimal quality of life on MDI)
- Indications at the clinical discretion of the health care professional (e.g. elevated HbA$_{1c}$ in type 2 diabetes treated by MDI)

General requirements:

- Motivated and willing to use CSII
- Willing to perform frequent blood glucose self-monitoring
- Ability to perform carbohydrate counting and insulin dosage adjustment
- Trained and capable of performing pump procedures

Relative contraindications:

- No team available to supervise CSII start and follow-up
- Unwilling or unable to perform pump procedures
- Significant psychiatric problems
- 'Brittle' diabetes

3.2 The patient pathway

Help in the organization, costing, and implementation of insulin pump services has been given in a recent UK report (Department of Health/Diabetes UK 2007) and costing template (NICE 2008b), and these can readily be adapted for use in other countries. We follow a sequential approach in adults who are candidates for CSII which targets pump therapy at those who remain poorly controlled on MDI (Figure 3.1) and where candidates for CSII are seen in turn:

- *By the physician.* Patients referred with difficult diabetes are probably best seen in a dedicated insulin pump clinic where the nature of the clinical problem is elicited, a diabetes and general medical history taken, physical examination performed as necessary, and blood and urine tests performed. The nature of CSII, its pros and cons, and the treatment plan are explained, and the patient is given an information pack about insulin pump therapy. If the physician and patient together consider that CSII is an option, patients are referred for:

- *A pre-pump assessment programme.* Here a diabetes specialist nurse and dietitian with expertise in CSII

  - assess the patient's existing knowledge and management of diabetes, and where necessary supervise renewed diabetes education in an attempt to optimize control on MDI. This includes attention to injection technique and sites, identification of lipohypertrophy, teaching of carbohydrate counting and treatment of hypoglycaemia, frequent blood glucose self-monitoring and insulin dosage adjustment and correcting doses, checking meter accuracy, and transfer to long-acting insulin analogues as necessary

  - discuss CSII with the patient in more detail, give a brief demonstration with regard to pumps and infusion sets, answer questions, and assess the patient's suitability for a trial of CSII

  - allow the patient time to discus the option of pump therapy at home with friends and relatives, and to decide if it is the right next approach for them. After this the patients are seen at

- *A second physician clinic visit.* Here the results of the pre-pump assessment, renewed education and actions taken are evaluated with the patient's views about CSII. Those who are now well controlled or decline CSII are returned to the normal diabetes clinic. Those who remain poorly controlled are offered a trial of CSII.

Note that many consider that in children with type 1 diabetes who remain poorly controlled on injection therapy, a trial of MDI is impractical (NICE 2008a) but a pre-pump programme is still valuable for detailed discussion of CSII (with parents and children), renewed education, and dietary input before proceeding to CSII.

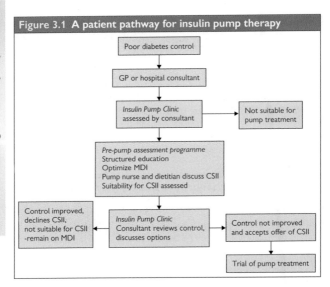

Figure 3.1 A patient pathway for insulin pump therapy

Poor diabetes control

GP or hospital consultant

Insulin Pump Clinic
assessed by consultant

Not suitable for
pump treatment

Pre-pump assessment programme
Structured education
Optimize MDI
Pump nurse and dietitian discuss CSII
Suitability for CSII assessed

Control improved,
declines CSII,
not suitable for CSII
-remain on MDI

Insulin Pump Clinic
Consultant reviews control,
discusses options

Control not improved
and accepts offer of CSII

Trial of pump treatment

3.3 **Starting insulin pump therapy**

3.3.1 **Choosing the initial insulin dosages of CSII (Figure 3.2)**

Monomeric insulin (lispro, aspart, or glulisine) is now regarded as the
pump insulin of choice, and dosages on pump therapy are estimated
as follows:

- *Basal rate*: A common starting approach is to reduce the total daily
  insulin dose on MDI by 20% (some centres reduce by 25%–30%).
  Give 50% of the pump total daily dose as a basal rate, divided by 24
  to give the hourly rate (Figure 3.2). Thus, a patient on 55 units
  insulin/day on MDI can be started on 80% of 55 units = 44 units
  insulin/day on CSII, and 44 ÷ 2 = 22 units/day at the basal rate.
  This is equivalent to 22 ÷ 24 = 0.9 units/hour. Use one basal rate
  throughout the day at first. Adjust the overnight basal rate by
  monitoring the fasting blood glucose (e.g. if the pre-breakfast
  blood glucose is higher than target, increase the basal rate by 0.05
  or 0.1 units/hour) and the 3 a.m. blood glucose (a normal 3 a.m.
  value and high pre-breakfast value would indicate a marked dawn
  phenomenon and the need for an increased basal rate from, say,
  3 a.m. to 9 a.m.). Adjust the daytime basal rate by missing a meal
  and monitoring blood glucose levels 2 hourly until just before the
  next meal (e.g. miss breakfast one day: a high blood glucose at
  1 pm indicating the need for an increased morning basal rate).

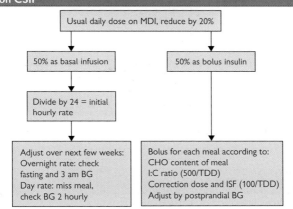

Figure 3.2 Choosing the initial basal and bolus insulin doses on CSII

- *Bolus insulin*: Originally, starting meal doses were calculated as 50% of the total CSII insulin dosage divided amongst the three main meals, often with proportionally more given for breakfast than its calorific content would suggest. In the above example, this represents 44 units ÷ 2 = 22 units/day for meals; say, 8 units at breakfast, 6 units at lunch, and 8 units at the evening meal. Bolus doses were then adjusted by measuring postprandial blood glucose concentrations (90min or 2 hours after the meal). Carbohydrate counting is now the preferred method (see Section 3.3.3), where bolus size is estimated according to the carbohydrate content of the meal, the insulin:carbohydrate ratio (I:C) for the individual and the meal, and a correction dose based on the pre-meal blood glucose level and how far it deviates from the target blood glucose concentration.

The I:C can be calculated as 500 ÷ total daily dose of insulin. This is often called 'the rule of 500', originally 'the rule of 450' when regular, short-acting insulin was used in the pump (Davidson *et al.* 2003). Round the I:C to the nearest 5. Thus, for a total dose of 44 units, I:C = 500 ÷ 44 = 11.5, which approximates to 1:10 (every 10g of carbohydrate at meals needs 1 unit of insulin).

The correction dose, used to adjust the meal bolus for the pre-meal blood glucose level and to correct unexpected hyperglycaemia between meals, is estimated by the insulin sensitivity factor (ISF), which for mmol/L is calculated as 100 ÷ the total daily insulin dose ('the rule of 100'). Thus, for the example used here, ISF = 100 ÷ 44 = 2.25, that is,

1 unit of insulin lowers the blood glucose concentration by about 2mmol/L. For mg/dL, the rule of 1800 (sometimes 1700) is used: 1800 ÷ 44 = 1 unit of insulin lowers the blood glucose by about 40mg/dL.

Box 3.2 shows an example of how the bolus is estimated for a meal of 60g carbohydrate, using the I:C ratio, pre-meal and target blood glucose, and ISF. There are recent suggestions from well-controlled patients on CSII with glucose levels monitored by continuous glucose monitoring that the bolus insulin dose calculated by these formulae may underestimate the amount of meal insulin needed (King and Armstrong 2007). However, we recommend using the I:C and ISF calculations given here and adjusting the insulin needed over the first weeks of CSII, using the blood glucose levels achieved postprandially in individual subjects (Figure 3.2).

Box 3.2 An example of estimation of the meal insulin bolus for CSII

Carbohydrate content of meal = 60g
I:C = 1:10 (for the case scenario)
ISF = 2.0
Pre-meal blood glucose = 8.0mmol/L
Target pre-meal blood glucose = 6.0mmol/L

Uncorrected bolus = 60 ÷ 10 = 6 units
Correction dose = (Pre-meal glucose − target glucose) ÷ ISF
$$= (8.0 - 6.0) ÷ 2.0 = 1 \text{ unit}$$
Therefore deliver for this meal via pump: 6 + 1 = 7 units of insulin.

3.3.2 The role of the dietitian in insulin pump therapy and shaping mealtime boluses

Dietitians play a crucial role in insulin pump therapy. Some patients can gain weight on switching to CSII as control improves, either because nutrients formerly lost in the urine in the poorly controlled state of MDI are now retained in the body or because the patient relaxes their food intake on CSII ('I can eat anything now')—see Chapter 4. The dietitian will need to work collaboratively with the patient to advise on a diet and exercise plan that enables good nutrition without excess weight gain, whilst maintaining dietary freedom.

Some patients are overweight or obese on MDI when they are referred for consideration of CSII, perhaps because they have been overeating to avoid or correct hypoglycaemia or because of over-insulinization on injection therapy. They may lose weight on transferring to CSII because of reduced hypoglycaemia and insulin requirements, but in those that maintain their overweight, suitable weight-reducing strategies should be discussed. Some patients starting CSII have existing cardiovascular disease (CVD) or risk factors for the development of CVD such as hypertension and hyperlipidaemia, and they will need particular dietary emphasis of the healthy eating plan appropriate for all—reduce saturated fats, low cholesterol, and low salt. It is important that these modifications are not seen as an additional burden but as a positive contribution to better health. Many patients need dietary advice about preventing hypoglycaemia: alcohol moderation or avoidance, appropriate use, and type of extra carbohydrate when exercising and when correcting unexpected hypoglycaemia.

However, a key task for the dietitian is the teaching of 'carbohydrate counting', really the matching of mealtime insulin dosage to food choice. This is now an integral part of all intensive insulin regimens, MDI as well as pump therapy, and a major component of structured education programmes such as DAFNE—Dosage Adjustment for Normal Eating—(DAFNE Study Group 2002). It is based on the assumption that the carbohydrate (CHO) content of meals has the most influence on the postprandial blood glucose, whilst noting that other aspects of meal composition also play a part:

- *Glycaemic index (GI)*—foods with a lower GI are digested and absorbed more slowly (and vice versa for high GI foods). Thus, pasta has a lower GI than mashed potato and may benefit from an extended square wave bolus during CSII. But judging the GI of foods is difficult, depending on food form, how it is cooked and processed, its acidity, the prevailing blood glucose and other factors, and most insulin pump patients do well even when omitting GI as a variable. The use of a measured amount of high GI carbohydrate as the treatment of choice for correcting hypoglycaemia is highly recommended.
- *Fat content*—high fat meals delay gastric emptying and cause late hyperglycaemia (but lower than expected blood glucose levels immediately after eating), and this may result in insulin resistance for 6–8 hours. An extended or square wave bolus might be helpful. Food diaries can be useful in helping the patient and dietitian identify where fat may be influencing blood glucose levels and hence where extended or square wave boluses may be useful.
- *Protein content*—high protein meals tend to have a delayed hyperglycaemic effect in some people with diabetes but accounting for protein is not usually necessary.

3.3.3 Carbohydrate counting

CHO counting is an essential element of pump therapy and is also recommended for MDI (see earlier). It offers a more precise and flexible approach to meal planning, and is about learning to adjust the insulin dose according to the type and amount of food chosen, and the different lifestyles and activity levels of individuals. CHO counting offers the patient the freedom to enjoy a variety of foods and to eat according to appetite.

Some patients will be familiar with the past practice of CHO counting in the form of 'exchanges'. In the exchange method of counting CHO, the patient is provided with a list of the portions or servings in different food groups that contain the same 10 or 15g exchange of CHO. For example, one portion of bread contains one 15g exchange. Vegetables are either not counted or given a 1/3 exchange. The exchange value differs in different countries, with either 15g or 10g lists being used. Although the patient can use the list with ease, as it does not require much skill in mathematics, it is not an exact way of counting CHO. Moreover, portion sizes have increased in recent years and what might have been one 15g or 10g exchange some decades ago is no longer the case. CHO counting in grams is now recommended for estimating meal content and adjusting insulin accordingly.

Patients may find CHO counting intimidating, confusing, and daunting at first. As with any new skill, CHO counting takes time and attention. It involves reading food labels and/or food reference books, recipes, measuring and weighing food (at least at first), and calculating the CHO in a meal, in addition to frequent blood glucose testing to determine the effect of the CHO on the blood glucose. This can seem a challenge but with structured and continuous education, and support from the dietitian, most patients master CHO counting reasonably well.

The following steps to counting CHO are useful:

- Identify foods containing CHO. CHO is found in bread, breakfast cereals, grains (pasta, rice, couscous), starchy vegetables (potato, yam, sweet potato), fruits, pulses, dairy, biscuits, pastries, cakes, and chocolate. There is some amount of CHO in alcohol but this needs to be counted with caution, in view of the hypoglycaemic effect of alcohol and the variable response to the quantity and type of alcohol.
- Calculate the CHO in the meal, using food labels or from the weight of the food. When reading food labels, it is important to pay attention to the suggested serving size and the serving size the patient actually consumes. The CHO = total weight of food/100 × CHO content of food per 100g of food (from food packaging or reference books).
- Determine the amount of CHO covered by 1 unit of insulin, the I:C ratio (see Section 3.3.1 for bolus insulin).

3.3.4 **Bolus calculators**

Most pumps have now become 'smart' in that they can calculate the bolus insulin based on input from the patient of the actual pre-meal and the target blood glucose levels, the intended carbohydrate intake in the meal, the I:C ratio, and the 'insulin on board' or active insulin (Zisser *et al.* 2008). The latter is the amount of insulin remaining from a previous bolus and is a concept designed to prevent 'stacking' or overestimation of meal insulin by ignoring the remaining insulin

---

Box 3.3 Checklist for CSII patient education

Pre-pump

What is insulin pump therapy, the rationale, advantages and disadvantages, best use, what is expected of pump user, how diabetes will be managed on pump, deciding if pump is right for patient, discussing with relatives and friends, demonstrating a pump, how a pump is worn, patient information leaflets, consider discussion with existing pump users, pump support groups

Pump initiation

Pump factors

Battery change

Pump operation, buttons, screen, programming, alarms

Basal rate, definition, set, alter, multiple rates and programmes, temporary basal and its uses

Bolus, definition, calculation, set, shapes, carbohydrate counting, I:C ratio, ISF

Insulin, type, load reservoir, connect infusion set, prime set

Cannula and infusion set, types, site selection, rotation, insertion, change and duration of use, quick release

Blood glucose self-monitoring and ketone testing

Target blood glucose values, HbA$_{1c}$ targets, frequency of testing, timing, recording, action, when to test for ketones and what to do

Pump life

How long-term pump therapy is followed up and supervised by healthcare team, hospital visits, and procedures

Exercise, sport, avoiding hypoglycaemia, and ketoacidosis

Travel, driving, sexual intimacy, menstrual cycle

Illness, stress, sick day rules, in-hospital use

Bathing, showering, swimming, pump rests

Troubleshooting, hyper- and hypoglycaemia, causes, correction doses

Pump malfunction, returning to MDI

Pump support groups

When and who to ask or call for help, manufacturer help lines, diabetes nurse/educator/dietitian, physician

and thus consequent hypoglycaemia. The calculations are different for different pumps, for example, some using curvilinear and some linear plots of per cent insulin remaining at times after administration. The duration of insulin action can either be varied or a default value can be used, which itself differs between pumps (3–6 hours). There are many sources of error in these calculations, including the established factors that can affect insulin absorption such as varying bolus size, environmental temperature, exercise, and individual variation in insulin absorption. Adjustments to the recommended bolus are therefore often needed and patients are wise to maintain the ability to calculate boluses manually, and it is common for patients to begin with manual estimates and to progress to integrated bolus calculators at a later stage. Whilst not suitable or used by all patients, bolus calculators have been found to reduce pre- and post-meal blood glucose levels and the number of correction doses needed compared to manual methods of bolus estimation (Shashaj *et al.* 2008).

3.3.5 **Starting CSII**

Thorough patient education is essential and begins before the pump start, at the stage of pre-pump assessment (Box 3.3). This is when a structured diabetes education programme is introduced, though many pump candidates have already done DAFNE-style courses (see Section 3.2); the rationale and pros and cons of CSII are also discussed, first patient questions answered and written information given. Targets for blood glucose control which are applicable to MDI and CSII (for the calculation of correction doses, see earlier) will be taught at this stage, and adjusted for the individual (lower in pregnancy, higher for hypoglycaemia unawareness at the start of CSII) (Table 3.1):

There are several models for starting patients on insulin pump therapy including group starts (more suitable at large centres with many potential pump candidates) and inpatient starts (more suitable for especially high-risk patients, e.g. pregnant diabetes), but a common method is an outpatient start with individual instruction and a week of saline in the pump with continued MDI, to get the patient safely used to the controls and procedures (Figure 3.3). One approach to pump starts (which we use) is to schedule two visits to the diabetes centre, one week apart, and arranging these for a Monday allows the first few days of CSII to be during the week rather than over a weekend. At visit 1, the pump nurse and dietitian institute first-line pump training; after the patient has used the pump at home with saline, training is continued at visit 2 and instructions given for reducing the long-acting insulin of MDI that night—a 50% reduction is usual. Switch to insulin in the pump can be made by the patient at home with daily telephone calls from the pump nurse for the first week and then at less frequent intervals (say, three per week in the second week and two per week in the third week after the start of CSII).

Table 3.1 Typical approximate target capillary blood glucose values

	Pre-meal	Postprandial	Bedtime
mmol/L	5–7	<10	6–8
mg/dL	90–130	<180	110–140

Figure 3.3 An example of a scheme for starting CSII as an outpatient

Pump nurse
2 hours, diabetes centre
Basic pump and cannula training
Calculate basal and bolus insulin
Given supplies, saline in pump

Pump dietitian
1 hour, diabetes centre
Revise CHO counting
Continue dietary education:
exercise, alcohol, weight control,
Follow-up as necessary

Patient at home for 1 week
Learns buttons, menus, do two set changes

Mon, 1 hour, diabetes centre
Reinforce training, review
Instructions for reducing long-acting insulin
Given contact numbers
Phone pump company, register, order supplies

Dietitan reviews/advises
as necessary

Tues, at home
Early switch to insulin in pump
Nurse phones at 5 pm, reviews BG, safety call at bedtime

Daily phone calls for 1 week
Thrice weekly calls for next week, adjust basal and bolus as necessary

3.3.6 Follow-up, audit, and long-term CSII

When good control is established on CSII, most patients need to be seen for follow-up in the hospital clinic at approximately 6 month intervals, that is, no more frequently than for MDI and in many cases much less frequently (because they are less troubled by hypo- and hyperglycaemia, and erratic control). One centre found that outpatient visits were reduced by 27% and admissions to hospital by 56% on CSII compared to MDI (Bruttomesso et al. 2002). It is usual at clinic visits to audit the effectiveness and potential complications of CSII by recording HbA$_{1c}$, weight/body mass index, frequency of severe hypoglycaemia, patterns in home blood glucose records, and to enquire about infusion site problems (infection, lipohypertrophy) and hospital admissions, as well as the normal checks of the diabetes clinic (blood pressure, tissue complications, lipids, etc.).

Many centres have patients who have used CSII and maintained excellent control for decades, and audits of clinics indicate that there is little or no deterioration in the mean HbA_{1c} of the pump population over many years (Bruttomesso *et al.* 2002). However, a few patients do not do well, either from the start or because they deteriorate after some months or years. Refresher courses might be helpful in some to remind patients of pump procedures and troubleshoot problems. But insulin pump therapy should not be continued unless the effectiveness can be demonstrated. The decision to revert to MDI in those who are clearly not benefiting is best made after discussion and agreement between the health care professionals and the patient or carer.

Most pumps now have the facility to download pump information to a computer or to the web for analysis (along with meter blood glucose and/or continuous glucose monitoring data, in some cases). Typical information includes basal delivery patterns and suspends, boluses given, pump alarms, carbohydrate given per meal, I:C and ISF used, and summary data such as mean blood glucose, high and low blood glucose, number of hypoglycaemic events, and mean total daily, basal and bolus insulin used. Such information is clearly valuable to the patient, physician, nurse, and dietitian in troubleshooting the reasons for poor control on the pump and optimizing pump treatment in general. Users of such downloaded information have lower HbA_{1c} values than non-users (Corriveau *et al.* 2008).

References

Blackett PR (1995). Insulin pump treatment for recurrent ketoacidosis in adolescence. *Diabetes Care*, **18**, 881–2.

Bruttomesso D, Pianta A, Crazzolara D *et al.* (2002). Continuous subcutaneous insulin infusion (CSII) in the Veneto region: efficacy, acceptability and quality of life. *Diabetic Medicine*, **19**, 628–34.

Corriveau EA, Durso PJ, Kaufman ED, Skipper BJ, Laskaratos LA, and Heintzman KB (2008). Effect of Carelink, an internet-based insulin pump monitoring system, on glycemic control in rural and urban children with type 1 diabetes mellitus. *Pediatric Diabetes*, **9**, 360–6.

DAFNE Study Group (2002). Training and flexible, intensive insulin management to enable dietary freedom in people with type 1 diabetes: dose adjustment for normal eating (DAFNE) randomised controlled trial. *British Medical Journal*, **325**, 746–56.

Davidson PC, Hebbelwhite HR, Bode BW *et al.* (2003). Statistically based CSII parameters: correction factor, CF (1700 rule), carbohydrate-to-insulin ratio, CIR (2.8 rule), and basal-to-total insulin ratio. *Diabetes Technology & Therapeutics*, **3**, 237.

Department of Health/Diabetes UK (2007). Insulin pump services: report of the Insulin Pump Working Group. Department of Health, London.

King AB and Armstrong DU (2007). A prospective evaluation of insulin dosage recommendations in patients with type 1 diabetes at near normal glucose control: bolus dosing. *Journal of Diabetes Science and Technology*, **1**, 42–6.

NICE (National Institute for Health and Clinical Excellence) (2008a). Continuous subcutaneous insulin infusion for the treatment of diabetes mellitus. Technology Appraisal Guidance 151 (Review of Technology Appraisal Guidance 57). NICE, London.

NICE (National Institute for Health and Clinical Excellence) (2008b). Continuous subcutaneous insulin infusion for the treatment of diabetes mellitus. Costing template and report. Implementing NICE Guidance. NICE, London.

Nielsen S, Kain D, Szudzik E, Dhindsa S, Garg R, and Dandona P (2005). Use of continuous subcutaneous insulin pump in patients with type 2 diabetes mellitus. *The Diabetes Educator*, **6**, 843–8.

Pickup JC and Hammond P (2009). NICE guidance on continuous subcutaneous insulin infusion 2008: review of the Technology Appraisal Guidance. *Diabetic Medicine*, **26**, 1–4.

Pickup JC, Williams G, Johns P, and Keen H (1983). Clinical features of brittle diabetic patients unresponsive to optimised subcutaneous insulin therapy (continuous subcutaneous insulin infusion). *Diabetes Care*, **6**, 279–84.

Schade DS, Drumm DA, Duckworth WC, and Eaton RP (1985). The etiology of incapacitating brittle diabetes. *Diabetes Care*, **8**, 12–20.

Shashaj B, Busetto E, and Sulli N (2008). Benefits of a bolus calculator in the pre- and postprandial glycaemic control and meal flexibility of paediatric patients using continuous subcutaneous insulin infusion (CSII). *Diabetic Medicine*, **25**, 1036–42.

Zisser H, Robinson L, Bevier W *et al.* (2008). Bolus calculator: a review of four 'smart' insulin pumps. *Diabetes Technology & Therapeutics*, **10**, 441–4.

Chapter 4

The pump life

Siobhan Pender, John Pickup

Key points

- Exercise-induced hypoglycaemia can be avoided during insulin pump therapy by taking extra carbohydrate, by reducing the bolus insulin (if exercise is within 2 hours of a meal), or by reducing the basal rate (for prolonged and/or intense exercise). Patients should not exercise if the blood glucose is greater than about 15mmol/L and there are ketones

- Bathing or showering is best done whilst the pump is temporarily disconnected from the infusion set, but waterproof pump cases can be used or the pump set on the bath side

- Pump use does not disturb sleep—it can be placed in the bed, on a bedside table, or worn

- Patients may chose to either wear the pump or disconnect it during sexual intimacy

- Pump rests for a few hours and are useful for sunbathing, sports, and medical procedures

- Insulin requirements often increase before menstruation, and the basal insulin rate should be increased at this time. A few women suffer hypoglycaemia, when the basal rate should be reduced

- Simple 'sick-day rules' are important for those on continuous subcutaneous insulin infusion (CSII); insulin requirements usually increase during illness; guidelines are available for continuing CSII as an inpatient

- Troubleshooting guides in the event of unexpected hypo- and hyperglycaemia on CSII are useful to detect problems and maintain strict glycaemic control

4.1 Exercise and sports

Exercise is an important component of diabetes management which should be employed and enjoyed by those using continuous subcutaneous insulin infusion (CSII) as much as insulin injection therapy. In type 1 diabetes, blood glucose levels tend to decrease if there is hyperinsulinaemia during exercise, or if the exercise is intensive or prolonged. Hypoglycaemia may be delayed for some 24–36 hours after the exercise and can be worse in those with hypoglycaemia unawareness and autonomic failure. On the other hand, strenuous exercise and the consequent production of counter-regulatory hormones can result in hyperglycaemia if blood insulin levels are low, and there can even be a risk of ketoacidosis.

4.1.1 **Avoiding hypoglycaemia with exercise**

If exercise is brief and moderate, and glycaemic control good at the start of exercise, usually no alterations in the pump regimen are necessary and control is maintained. The simplest strategy to avoid hypoglycaemia when exercise is mild or moderate is to consume extra carbohydrate, about 30–60g for each hour of activity (30g before and each 30min point), and to monitor blood glucose before and after the exercise, and to check for late hypoglycaemia. This approach is recommended in the first months after starting CSII whilst patients are learning the basics of pump therapy. An alternative estimation of the required extra carbohydrate is 1g/kg body weight/hour (Perkins and Ridell 2006). Athletes and keen sportsmen can also refer to tables which relate the type of sport and body weight to the extra carbohydrate needed per hour of activity (Perkins and Ridell 2006).

Reducing insulin dosage is a more complicated strategy to avoid hypoglycaemia but is more likely to encourage weight loss with exercise. If exercise is within 2 hours of a meal and bolus, the bolus insulin dose should be reduced; the amount of reduction can be calculated from the extra carbohydrate needed and the carbohydrate:insulin ratio for the subject. For example, if 60g of carbohydrate is estimated as needed and the C:I is 1:15, then the bolus should be reduced by 4 units.

For prolonged and intense exercise, or activity remote from mealtimes, a reduction in the basal insulin rate is recommended, usually varying from 10% to 50%, and beginning 90min before exercise starts and continuing for 90min after the end of exercise. For contact sports, special pump cases are available from manufacturers that guard against pump damage and hold the pump securely during the sport. Many prefer to remove the pump, best done by disconnecting the cannula at the infusion set, rather than suspending the pump (which might encourage insulin blockage in the cannula). Glycaemic control tends to be stable for about 1 hour after stopping infusion (Pickup et al. 1982), but longer periods of pump disconnect require a supplemental injection of insulin when CSII is resumed—say, 50% of the insulin dose that would have been infused.

For regular sportsmen where the pump will be disconnected for 2 hours or so on a frequent basis, some recommend the option of (whilst continuing with CSII) injecting a small dose of long-acting insulin at bedtime, such as glargine, and reducing the pump basal rate appropriately. This ensures that during pump disconnect background insulin will be supplied by the injected insulin.

4.1.2 Avoiding hyperglycaemia and ketosis with exercise

If the blood glucose level is greater than about 15mmol/L, the subject should check for ketones. Exercise should not be performed when there is ketosis, a correction insulin dose should be administered and exercise delayed until ketones are absent. When the blood glucose is >15mmol/L without ketones (e.g. after a meal with insufficient bolus insulin), exercise may be undertaken.

4.2 Bathing, showering, hot tubs, and saunas

Patient questions

- Can the insulin pump get wet?
- How will I shower? Can I remove the insulin pump when I shower?
- Will I no longer be able to have a bath?
- Can I take my pump into a sauna?

Although a number of pumps are now waterproof or water resistant (and some are not), the pump should not be put directly in water and it is best to avoid the pump and its electronic components getting wet. Bathing and showering can be accomplished in three ways: the infusion set can be disconnected from the cannula with a quick-release mechanism, a protective cap placed on the connector and pump and the pump set aside; a waterproof plastic bag or other protective case supplied by the pump manufacturer can be used to protect the pump (say, hung around the shower head or around the user's neck); or the pump can be placed on side of the bath (this is not recommended because of the danger of the pump falling in the water). Most pump users disconnect for up to 1 hour when bathing or showering. To avoid forgetting to restart the pump following reconnection after showering/bathing, the user is encouraged to leave the pump running.

Although some pumps may be waterproof, immersing them in or exposing them to very hot water or steam (like a Jacuzzi or sauna) is not recommended. High heat may reduce insulin potency and exposing a pump or infusion line in this way can result in hyperglycaemia or ketoacidosis. Heat may also increase subcutaneous insulin absorption and increase the risk of hypoglycaemia when bathing after a bolus. For these reasons, we recommend that pumps are best disconnected for bathing and showering. To identify unexpected hypoglycaemia and hyperglycaemia, the pump user should monitor blood glucose frequently following bathing.

4.3 Sleeping

Patient questions
• How can I sleep with the pump?
• Will I pull the cannula out at night?
• Will the pump keep me awake?

Worrying about how to sleep with an insulin pump is common for new pump users. Individuals are nervous about the pump interfering with their regular sleeping habits or the infusion set becoming disconnected during sleep. There may be anxiety about not being in control of the technology during this time or by being woken by alarms.

Some insulin pump wearers place their insulin pump next to them on the bed, while others put it in a pocket in their pyjamas. Placing the insulin pump under their pillow is a popular option as it is easy to locate. Most pump users report no discomfort whilst sleeping and wearing the pump and it is rare for the infusion set to dislodge whilst sleeping. Activating the key lock during sleep will avoid the user from accidentally giving a bolus. Most modern pumps are virtually silent during operation and do not disturb sleep because of noise.

A wide range of pump accessories, which are useful during sleep, are available, including long infusion set tubing (which allows the pump to be placed on a bedside table), neck ribbons, and soft belts.

The patient will be further reassured about wearing the pump at night by explaining that the pump provides a continuous background supply of insulin throughout the night, as well as the day, allowing the user to sleep in and miss or delay breakfast without risking morning hyperglycaemia, and allowing preprogrammed changes in basal insulin rates in the sleeping hours to prevent night-time hypoglycaemia or pre-breakfast hyperglycaemia.

4.4 **Sexual intimacy**

Patient questions

• What should I do with the insulin pump during sex?
• Will my partner reject me because of the pump?

Most insulin pump users are concerned about this initially, and may not feel comfortable broaching the subject with their clinician. The subject should be discussed as part of the insulin pump pre-assessment (Chapter 3). Insulin pump therapy is less likely to impact on sexual intimacy if it is discussed openly with both the patient and his/her partner. Partners and potential partners who accept a patient's diabetes as a whole usually have no issues with an insulin pump and its place in the life of the patient (Farkas-Hirsch and Hirsch 1994).

If both partners are comfortable with the insulin pump, it can be left in place during sexual intimacy. The infusion cannula can get pulled during sexual activity, but it should be explained that this is not harmful, though the positioning of the infusion set should be checked carefully before falling asleep to ensure the system is still intact. In many cases, the patient will decide to disconnect the pump during periods of intimacy, particularly when planning for a change of cannula and infusion set afterwards (Farkas-Hirsch and Hirsch 1994); when this disconnection lasts longer than 1 hour, an insulin replacement injection or bolus via the pump will be needed. The pump user should avoid falling asleep before the pump is replaced.

4.5 **Temporarily removing the insulin pump—pump rests**

43

Patient questions

• What do I do if I want to have some time off the pump?
• I don't want to sunbathe with a pump on.
• I will be water skiing all day and my pump is not waterproof—what do I do?

Temporary pump 'rests' are part of the normal, planned pump regimen and are useful for bathing and showering, contact and water sports, and sexual intimacy, as discussed earlier, and also for sunbathing and medical procedures such as X-ray, computer tomography (CT), and magnetic resonance imaging (MRI). Pump malfunction might lead to a more extended break until the pump can be replaced.

If glycaemic control is reasonable, nothing needs to be done for the first hour of disconnect, when control is maintained (Pickup *et al.* 1982). For longer periods of time, such as a day at the beach and water sports, short-acting insulin (regular or monomeric) can be given as bolus injections at mealtimes during the disconnect (perhaps a little augmented to cover the absent basal insulin), and combined with frequent blood glucose self-monitoring to check control. (Keep the pump and cannula out of the sunlight when at the beach, for example, by putting a towel over the pump to shade it or putting the pump in an insulin cool bag). For an overnight pump rest, a bedtime injection of intermediate-acting insulin (isophane, lente, or detemir) is best to cover the basal supply, and for longer pump absences of a day or more, reverting to multiple dose insulin injections will be required—twice daily intermediate-acting insulin or daily glargine, with short-acting insulin at meals. The patient will have been given clear instructions about how to return to injection therapy during pump training (Chapter 3).

4.6 **Menses**

Patient questions

• I always have high blood glucose tests a few days before my period starts? What can I do to control my blood glucose levels?
• The insulin I bolus for my carbohydrate appears to have little effect.
• Once my period starts, I experience hypoglycaemia.

Glycaemic control and insulin requirements alter in about half of women before and around the time of menstruation, most needing more insulin, but some 10% need less. Insulin pump therapy can help women reduce blood glucose excursions at the time of menses. Most women with diabetes are keen to know how best to manage their diabetes before, during, and after their menstrual cycle and should be given specific instructions. An increase in the basal rate is the usual need at the time of pre-menstrual hyperglycaemia, say starting with an increase of 0.1 unit/hour, and returning to the normal basal rate after menstruation. This menstrual basal rate profile can be programmed into many pumps. For those few who suffer from hypoglycaemia at the time of menstruation, a reduction of 0.1 unit/hour may be tried as a first measure.

4.7 Illness and stress

Patient questions

- How do I manage the insulin pump when I'm ill?
- Will I need to go back onto insulin injections?
- If I'm unable to look after my insulin pump when I'm ill, what should I do?
- If I go into hospital who will look after my insulin pump?
- Will I have to remove my insulin pump if I'm admitted to hospital?

4.7.1 Sick day rules

Illness such as infections and injury, as well as severe emotional stress can frequently lead to hyperglycaemia and, sometimes, ketoacidosis in type 1 diabetes. Pump users are at potential risk because, with the increased demands of illness and the subcutaneous insulin depot being smaller than during injection therapy, ketosis may develop quickly. Interestingly, however, many studies have shown that the frequency of diabetic ketoacidosis is about the same during CSII and injection therapy (Bending *et al.* 1985; Chantelau *et al.* 1989; Bode *et al.* 1996; Boland *et al.* 1999), indicating that with proper education, careful monitoring, and attention to guidelines on illness manage-ment, patients are not at an actual increased risk. In general, 'sick day rules' are similar to those used for other people with type 1 diabetes, but clear and simple instructions are necessary during pump training (Chapter 3), and are especially useful for patients who will not be at their most proactive and clear-thinking state during illness or stress (Box 4.1).

Sick-day rules are usually effective in lowering blood glucose levels and clearing ketones but the health care team should be contacted if hyperglycaemia persists, ketones do not resolve, or vomiting occurs. Clinicians must ensure that patients have in-date ketone strips and access to insulin syringes or insulin pen devices. The basal rate usu-ally needs to be increased by 30%–100% during infections, depending on the severity of the illness—colds might need 50% increase and chest infections 100%. The basal rate may need increasing for tempo-rary emotional stress lasting some days or weeks (say bereavement), but the hyperglycaemic effect of short-term stress (giving a speech) can be countered with a correction bolus.

> **Box 4.1 Simple sick-day rules for those on insulin pump therapy**
>
> - Monitor blood glucose more frequently and test for ketones if feeling unwell
> - If blood glucose >15 mmol/L on more than two occasions, check for ketones
> - If ketones not present—usual correction dose may be used
> - If ketones present—give extra insulin by syringe or pen (correction dose plus 50%), check pump and infusion set
> - If there is doubt about insulin pump delivery, replace the reservoir and infusion set, using a new infusion set and new insulin
> - Basal insulin rate may need increasing 30%–100% for duration of illness (temporary basal rate feature may be used)
> - When blood glucose elevated, increase fluid intake with non-calorific drinks to avoid dehydration
> - Do not stop insulin when ill—continue basal insulin, even if not eating, or if vomiting and not giving boluses
> - When blood glucose returns to near-normal, carbohydrates will be necessary to clear ketones (a snack and appropriate bolus)
> - Contact diabetes team if high blood glucose levels, ketones, or vomiting continue; if self-care is difficult or well-being deteriorates; or if you are uncertain how to manage the situation

4.7.2 **Continuing CSII in hospital**

Most pump users will wish to continue CSII during a hospital admission but they may be concerned about transferring their care to staff who they perceive as knowing less about pump procedures than they do. Clearly, many health care professionals will not be experts in CSII and many hospitals will not have access to pump supplies, so patients can expect that they will often be switched to insulin injection therapy. However, guidelines have been prepared for those hospitals allowing the continuation of pump use during an admission (Box 4.2) (Cook *et al.* 2005).

4.7.3 **CSII and minor surgery and investigations**

The pump user should discuss the nature of the medical procedures and how their diabetes will be managed before surgery with the admitting doctor and if appropriate the anaesthetist. For minor operations not requiring a general anaesthetic, the pump may be continued at the basal rate, and correction doses used to maintain glycaemic control as necessary. It will be necessary to remove the pump for X-ray, CT, or MRI scans, and a pump rest of 1 hour will not cause any metabolic disruption (see Section 4.5). Frequent blood glucose monitoring after the procedure will identify any hyper- or hypoglycaemia.

Box 4.2 Requirements for continuing CSII as an inpatient

Patients should be:

- Alert and orientated
- Willing to continue CSII and willing to sign a consent form and adhere to any hospital requirements (e.g. inform staff of boluses and basal rates used, pump problems, hypoglycaemia experienced, provide supplies, recognize the need to discontinue CSII on doctor's orders, etc.)
- Not incapable through cognitive or motor impairments of undertaking pump procedures
- Not critically ill/requiring intensive care
- Not considered a suicide risk
- Able to supply pump and consumables
- Willing to allow a family member/friend to assist if patient unable to manage CSII, and providing such person is pump-trained and remains with the patient at all times

4.7.4 **CSII and major surgery**

The usual practice for all people with type 1 diabetes and those with insulin-requiring type 2 diabetes who are undergoing significant surgery is to control the diabetes with intravenous infusion of insulin and glucose infusion, and this also should be the case in pump users. As it takes several hours to reach the intended steady-state blood insulin levels after commencing CSII at the basal rate (Chapter 1), the insulin pump should be recommenced with a basal rate 10%–20% higher than usual some 4 hours before discontinuing the intravenous insulin infusion.

4.8 **Travel**

Patient questions

- Can I travel abroad with my insulin pump?
- What do I need to pack in my travel hand luggage?
- What do I need to do if travelling through time zones?

Pump users who travel should have documentation detailing their need to wear an insulin pump and to carry insulin, supplies, and equipment. A travel bag should contain insulin, infusion sets, reservoirs, syringes/pens, blood glucose monitoring strips and meters, snacks and water, and should be taken on-board a plane as hand luggage or kept with the patient on other journeys such as by train.

Insulin should not be put in the hold of a plane where freezing temperatures may affect the stability of the insulin.

If travelling through time zones, the clock on the pump should be changed to the local time.

4.9 **Potential pump problems**

4.9.1 **Troubleshooting high and low blood glucose levels**

It is useful to have a check list for the patient and the health care professional, which will help them to identify the cause of unexpected hyperglycaemia or hypoglycaemia (Box 4.3).

Box 4.3 Troubleshooting unexpected hyperglycaemia
Check for hyperglycaemia due to:
Cannula problems
• Disconnected/leaking at infusion site or pump
• Cannula kinked
• Cannula blocked
• Air in system
• Failure to prime after changing the infusion set
Infusion site problems
• Infection, inflammation
• Lipohypertrophy
• Leaking at site
• Infusion set dislodged
• Infusion set used for >3 days
Pump malfunction/insulin problems
• Low battery (alarm would sound)
• Inadequate insulin in reservoir (alarm would sound)
• Insulin reservoir improperly placed in pump
• Insulin past expiration date
• Insulin inactive because of freezing or warmth
• Mechanical/electrical failure of pump (alarm would sound)
Patient problems
• Forgotten bolus
• Low bolus or misjudged carbohydrate
• Incorrect basal rates
• Over-correction with carbohydrate of hypoglycaemia
• Illness, emotional stress, inactivity increasing insulin requirements
• Drugs (e.g. steroids)
• Menstruation, pregnancy increasing insulin requirements

4.9.2 **Weight gain**

As with the institution of any regimen of strict glycaemic control in the previously poorly controlled individual with diabetes, there is a danger of weight gain when CSII is started, and several audits of long-term CSII have confirmed a modest weight increase (Bruttomesso *et al.* 2002). However, we have found that on average, insulin pump therapy is weight neutral in the patients in our insulin pump clinic, with the weight in some patients increasing, some decreasing, and some remaining fairly stable during the duration of CSII. Hypoglycaemia-prone patients are often overweight on MDI because they are over-insulinized on injections, may be snacking frequently to avoid hypoglycaemia and avoiding exercise which they know will worsen hypoglycaemia. Insulin pump therapy can help to reduce weight in these patients, because of the need for less insulin per day on CSII, the reduced frequency of hypoglycaemia allows the patient to take less extra food and exercise without hypoglycaemia can be promoted more easily on the pump (Box 4.4).

Nevertheless, advice from the pump dietitian is essential to avoid either weight gain or the maintenance of overweight when patients are switched to CSII (Chapter 3). In particular:

- Avoid the patient overeating as a consequence of a new-found dietary freedom ('I can now eat what I like'). Healthy eating should be instituted and maintained in the pump patient as in everyone else.
- Calories which were formerly lost in the urine as glycosuria in the poorly controlled subject are retained in the well-controlled patient on CSII, and weight gain will result unless the patient adjusts his diet appropriately and with the help of the dietitian.

Box 4.4 Troubleshooting unexpected hypoglycaemia

- Bolus insulin dose too much for food intake
- Excessive boluses being used to correct hyperglycaemia
- Basal rate too much for requirements
- Exercise without extra carbohydrate, or reduced bolus/basal insulin
- Delayed effect of exercise
- Target levels set too low by patient or doctor
- Alcohol intake
- Gastroparesis (delayed gastric emptying and mismatch of bolus insulin and food absorption)
- Infrequent blood glucose self-monitoring (does not allow patient to detect trends in glycaemia and to identify and correct impending hypoglycaemia)

4.9.3 **Infusion site problems**

Infection of the infusion site is now uncommon. Although probably more frequent than with injection therapy, the risk is reduced by limiting the duration of cannula use to 3 days, not re-using cannulae and employing a no-touch technique for insertion. When infection does occur, it is confined to the subcutaneous tissue, and even when notable it is more often a cellulitis rather than an abscess (Lenhard and Reeves 2001). It is usually easily dealt with. Organisms reported include *Staphylococcus aureus*, *S. epidermidis*, and *Mycobacterium fortuitum*. The infusion set should be removed, discarded, and another site and set used. Oral antibiotics are usually given but topical antibiotics are effective in early infections. Occasionally, a subcutaneous abscess needs surgical lancing. Irritation at the infusion site can be the result of contact dermatitis from infusion set components and tape, or due to friction. It is very unusual that its severity causes CSII to be stopped. The commonest cause of poor tape adhesion is sweating, and often antiperspirant applied to the skin and allowed to dry is helpful.

Lipohypertrophy occurs when insulin is infused into the same site over a period of time, just as it does when insulin injections are given into the same subcutaneous site. It results in impaired and erratic insulin absorption and is a notable cause of suboptimal glycaemic control. Patients should be educated as to the need for rotation of infusion sites (Chapter 3). Examination for lipohypertrophy and advising the patient to use a new site is sometimes successful in improving control in those poorly controlled on CSII, particularly those with worsening control after initial success with pump therapy.

References

Bending JJ, Pickup JC, and Keen H (1985). Frequency of diabetic ketoacidosis and hypoglycemic coma during treatment with continuous subcutaneous insulin infusion. *The American Journal of Medicine*, **79**, 685–91.

Bode BW, Steed RD, and Davidson PC (1996). Reduction in severe hypoglycemia with long-term continuous subcutaneous insulin infusion in type 1 diabetes. *Diabetes Care*, **19**, 324–7.

Boland EA, Grey M, Oesterle A, Fredrickson L, and Tamborlane WV (1999). Continuous subcutaneous insulin infusion. A new way to lower risk of severe hypoglycemia, improve metabolic control, and enhance coping in adolescents with type 1 diabetes. *Diabetes Care*, **22**, 1779–84.

Bruttomesso D, Pianta A, and Crazzolara D (2002). Continuous subcutaneous insulin infusion (CSII) in the Veneto region: efficacy, acceptability and quality of life. *Diabetic Medicine*, **19**, 628–34.

Chantelau E, Spraul M, Mühlhauser I, Gause R, and Berger M (1989). Long-term safety, efficacy and side effects of continuous subcutaneous insulin infusion treatment for type 1 (insulin-dependent) diabetes mellitus: a one centre experience. *Diabetologia*, **32**, 421–6.

Cook CB, Boyle ME, and Cisar NS (2005). Use of continuous subcutaneous insulin infusion (insulin pump) therapy in the hospital setting. *The Diabetes Educator*, **31**, 849–57.

Farkas-Hirsch R and Hirsch IB (1994). Continuous subcutaneous insulin infusion: review of the past and its implementation for the future. *Diabetes Spectrum*, **7**, 80–138.

Lenhard MJ and Reeves GD (2001). Continuous subcutaneous insulin infusion. A comprehensive review of insulin pump therapy. *Archives of Internal Medicine*, **161**, 2293–300.

Perkins BA and Riddell MC (2006). Type 1 diabetes and exercise: using the insulin pump to maximum advantage. *Canadian Journal of Diabetes*, **30**, 72–9.

Pickup JC, Viviberti GC, and Bilous RW (1982). Safety of continuous subcutaneous insulin infusion: metabolic deterioration and glycaemic autoregulation after deliberate cessation of infusion. *Diabetologia*, **22**, 175–9.

Chapter 5

CSII and continuous glucose monitoring in children and adolescents

Tadej Battelino

> ## Key points
>
> - Continuous subcutaneous insulin infusion (CSII) and real-time continuous glucose monitoring (RT-CGM) is safe, feasible, and effective in all age groups
> - Most infants, toddlers, children, and adolescents are eligible candidates
> - Thorough education and monitoring of patients, families, and caregivers are paramount
> - CSII significantly increases patients' flexibility and quality of life
> - RT-CGM improves metabolic control without increasing the risk of hypoglycaemia

5.1 Introduction

Despite the successful introduction of short- and long-acting insulin analogues and frequent self blood glucose (BG) monitoring with multiple daily injections, young people with diabetes, their families, and their diabetes care providers continue to struggle with everyday metabolic control. Recommended age-appropriate levels of glycated haemoglobin (HbA$_{1c}$) are achieved in only a minority of cases. In addition, the quality of life of young people with diabetes is compromised by an unpleasant daily routine, fear of hypoglycaemia, and various influences from their peers. Finally, adolescence, with its hormonal and behavioural peculiarities, accelerates the progression of chronic complications of diabetes and substantially reduces the compliance of this patient group. It is therefore understandable that the help of technology in the form of modern insulin pumps and real-time continuous glucose monitoring (RT-CGM) have gained increasing popularity in young people with diabetes. Continuous subcutaneous insulin infusion

(CSII) is becoming the predominant routine treatment modality in several large centres for paediatric diabetes around the globe.

5.2 **Clinical evidence**

Only a handful of randomized controlled clinical trials (RCTs) with limited numbers of patients in the paediatric age group have compared multiple daily insulin injections (MDI) utilizing modern insulin analogues with CSII. Most of them have demonstrated an equal effectiveness of MDI and CSII regarding HbA$_{1c}$, but significant superiority of CSII over MDI regarding severe hypoglycaemia, ketoacidosis (DKA), and quality of life (QoL). A recent meta-analysis of RCTs in paediatrics reports a significant decrease of HbA$_{1c}$ by 0.4% in patients using CSII, as compared to those using MDI. Several follow-up reports from centres of paediatric diabetes show significantly improved metabolic control and a reduction of acute complications with CSII over several years. Considering the difficulties with injecting insulin in infants and toddlers, CSII offers an effective mode of insulin delivery with considerably less parental stress. Moreover, CSII increases flexibility of lifestyle, especially that related to various physical activities. In the United Kingdom, NICE (National Institute for Health and Clinical Excellence) now recommends CSII as a treatment option for children and adolescents aged 12 years or older with type 1 diabetes in whom MDI has caused disabling hypoglycaemia when achieving the target HbA$_{1c}$ has been attempted, or when HbA$_{1c}$ levels have remained high ($\geq$8.5%) during MDI therapy (NICE 2008). CSII is also recommended in children less than 12 years of age whenever the use of MDI is impractical or inappropriate (see Chapter 3). Hence, CSII is currently considered the most physiological treatment modality for type 1 diabetes, and is preferred by an increasing number of young people with this type of diabetes.

5.3 **Patient selection**

The decision to begin CSII is ideally taken jointly by the child, parent(s)/guardians, and the diabetes team. Common clinical indications for CSII are summarized in Box 5.1. Several additional situations may prompt the suggestion of starting CSII, including feeding difficulties, adolescent rebellious non-compliance, co-morbidity, certain types of disability (e.g. cerebral palsy), and others. In routine clinical practice, most children and adolescents will meet criteria for initiating CSII, with some criteria being more prevalent in specific age groups.

CSII may be initiated at diagnosis in neonates, infants, toddlers, and children. If the remission phase is pronounced and the insulin requirement very low, starting CSII at the end of remission may be more appropriate.

Box 5.1 The indications for CSII in children and adolescents

Strong indications

- Recurrent severe hypoglycaemia
- Neonates, infants, toddlers, and preschool children
- Suboptimal diabetes control (i.e. HbA_{1c} exceeding target for age)
- Wide fluctuations in BG levels regardless of HbA_{1c}
- A pronounced dawn phenomenon
- Microvascular complications and/or risk factors for macrovascular complications
- Ketosis-prone individuals
- Good metabolic control but an insulin regimen that compromises lifestyle

Other indications

- Adolescents with eating disorders
- Children with needle phobia
- Insulin dose omissions
- Pregnant adolescents, ideally during preconception

5.4 Technology selection

Several technologically advanced insulin pump models are currently available. Favourable technical characteristics are summarized in Box 5.2.

Integrated bolus calculators that determine an insulin dose based on the preset insulin-to-carbohydrate ratio and insulin sensitivity may be particularly helpful if the dose is determined by a secondary caregiver like grandparents or school personnel. Some pump models receive and display data from an integrated RT-CGM device that may further improve beneficial results of the CSII treatment (see Chapter 8).

Box 5.2 Favourable technical characteristics for insulin pumps

- Flexible basal rate adjustment with the option of 0.05, 0.025, or 0.01 U/hr (for newborn, infants, toddlers)
- Flexible bolus insulin options with composite boluses (e.g. 'dual bolus')
- Adjustable alarms with 'reminders'
- Integrated bolus calculators
- Direct communication with a home BG meter
- Integrated tables with food choices and carbohydrate 'counts'
- Downloadable to a personal computer and/or uploadable to the web
- Integrated RT-CGM device

The ultimate choice of insulin pump is made preferably by the patient and/or primary caregiver, as personal attitude towards the device may influence its use, particularly in adolescents.

Catheter selection depends on patient age, activity, and personal preferences. A shorter subcutaneous catheter (length 6–8 mm) may be preferable in children with less subcutaneous fat, sometimes with an insertion angle <90°. Conversely, longer subcutaneous catheters are necessary in adolescents (length 9mm or more) to minimize catheter dislodgement. Shorter tubing is safer for children and longer usually preferred by adolescents, with an easy option for disconnecting at the insertion site.

Insulin selection remains with the three currently registered fast-acting insulin analogues: aspart (NovoRapid®), lispro (Humalog®), and glulisine (Apidra®), with basically comparable safety and efficacy.

5.5 **Structured educational programme**

The importance of thorough education of the patient, family, and possibly secondary caregivers cannot be overemphasized (Chapter 3). A team including a paediatric diabetologist, a specialized nurse educator, and a dietitian may provide the best mix for the structured information that is indispensable for successful CSII treatment. We consider that all education is preferably provided in an outpatient setting. Frequent re-education in specific topics is often required for sustained improvement of metabolic control (Box 5.3). Optimally, patients and caregivers should be able to contact a health care professional frequently and on a 24-hour availability basis.

> **Box 5.3 Structured educational programmes for CSII in children and adolescents**
>
> **These should include:**
> - A short background on the importance of good metabolic control
> - Principles of basal-bolus insulin therapy based on self BG monitoring
> - Food selection with carbohydrate counting (including notes on protein and fat)
> - Technical features of the chosen insulin pump, including catheter insertion
> - Principles of basal insulin rate selection (including temporary basal)
> - Principles of calculating meal and correction boluses
> - Recognition and management of hypoglycaemia and hyperglycaemia/DKA
> - Management of activity and exercise
> - Management of sick days

Patients and/or caregivers are encouraged to take the initiative and responsibility for managing diabetes with CSII. Several additional aspects are discussed with patients and/or caregivers according to specific needs and circumstances (e.g. the possibility of excessive weight gain, the question of the 'visibility' of the insulin pump, with practical suggestions of where to put it on various occasions, the question of travelling with an insulin pump, summer camps, etc.). Education in small groups (two to three families) may be more motivating.

5.6 Initiating CSII

A 3- to 5-day CGM recording can be used to determine patient-specific glucose fluctuations immediately before the CSII initialization. Alternatively, patients and/or caregivers may be asked to measure blood glucose 6–8 times daily 3 days before starting CSII. In both cases, a detailed logbook which includes the patient's habits and activities at the time of glucose monitoring is helpful.

Long-acting insulin or insulin analogues are omitted on the evening before the day of CSII initiation, and glycaemic control maintained as necessary by short-acting insulin. After the patient and caregiver have acquired all necessary knowledge and skills, the CSII insulin dose distribution is determined and CSII started with the first catheter insertion under the supervision of the health care professional.

5.6.1. Setting the basal insulin rate

Assuming that the patient has been in reasonable control on MDI, a reduction of the total daily dose (TDD) for CSII is recommended (see also Chapter 3). The percentage reduction increases with higher TDDs. An average of 10%–15% reduction is usually sufficient in infants, toddlers, and pre-school children, whereas a 20%–25% reduction may be warranted in insulin-resistant adolescents. Somewhat less than 50% of the reduced TDD is usually recommended for the basal rate.

The distribution of the basal rate varies significantly with age (Boxes 5.4 and 5.5). A constant basal rate is commonly required in pre-school children, with a possible modest increase in the basal requirement before midnight. With puberty, the basal rate evolves towards the typical dual rate requirements of young adults, with an increase in early morning and late afternoon (to cover for the 'dawn' and 'dusk phenomena').

Box 5.4 Setting the basal insulin rate for a 3-year-old girl (body weight 15kg, TDD on MDI 11 units)

- Reduction of TDD by 10% is 11 − 1 = 10U/day
- Up to 50% used for the basal rate = up to 5U/day
- Mean basal rate = 5 ÷ 24 = 0.2U/hr
- Recommended basal rate distribution:

Time	Basal rate (U/hr)	Total (U)
0–6	0.1	0.6
6–12	0.25	1.5
12–20	0.20	1.6
20–24	0.15	0.6
24 hours total		**4.3***

* It is prudent to start with a slightly lower basal rate to avoid hypoglycaemia.

In neonates, infants, and toddlers where the TDD on CSII is below 8 units, a basal rate <0.1U/hr is necessary. Some older insulin pump models do not have an option of lower basal rates and clogging of insulin in the catheter may increase in some patients with very low basal rates. Diluting insulin 1:1 or 1:10 with a diluent provided by the manufacturer or with normal sterile saline is an option employed by many parents in several centres of paediatric diabetes. However, newer insulin pump models allow for a basal rate of 0.025 or even 0.01U/hr, which greatly facilitates management of very low insulin requirements. In addition, the basal rate can be set to zero for 30–60min if hypoglycaemia occurs despite the low basal rate.

In adolescents, the dawn phenomenon is rather frequent and a high basal rate may be required to cover it. The dusk phenomenon is less frequent and usually requires a lower basal rate than that used to counter the dawn phenomenon. Most children and adolescents need a higher basal rate in the morning during school days, as compared to the weekend (a separate basal rate for the weekend may be set and stored in the insulin pump). Every basal rate is typically individual and must be tailored to the specific needs of each patient (Boxes 5.4 and 5.5).

5.6.2 **Verifying and adjusting the basal rate**

There is a requirement for basal insulin changes with the growth of the patient and during various periods of the school year. Patients are encouraged to verify the basal rate every 4–6 weeks on days with no extraordinary events and with starting BG values between 5 and 10mmol/L. For the morning profile, they omit breakfast and the morning snack and check the BG every 2 hours until lunch; for the afternoon profile, they omit lunch and the afternoon snack and measure the BG until dinner; and for the night profile, they eat a light

> ## Box 5.5 Setting the basal insulin rate for a 14-year-old pubertal boy (body weight 67kg, TDD on MDI 60 units)
>
> - Reduction of TDD by 20% = 60 − 12 = 48U/day
> - Up to 50% used for the basal rate = up to 24U/day
> - Mean basal rate = 24 ÷ 24 = 1.0U/hr
> - Recommended basal rate distribution:
>
> | Time | Basal rate (U/hr) | Total (U) |
> |------|-------------------|-----------|
> | 0–4 | 0.7 | 2.8 |
> | 4–7 | 1.3 | 3.9 |
> | 7–13 | 1.1 | 6.6 |
> | 13–20 | 1.0 | 7.0 |
> | 20–24 | 0.8 | 3.2 |
> | **24 hours total** | | **23.5*** |
>
> * It is prudent to start with a slightly lower basal rate to avoid hypoglycaemia.

early dinner at 5 p.m. and measure the BG throughout the night. The same procedure can be conveniently performed by a CGM device. When the BG does not remain stable within ±2mmol/L, appropriate adjustments of the basal rate are recommended. In smaller children, one meal at a time can only be omitted and more consecutive days are needed to verify the basal rate. Alternatively, a standard meal with a well-determined insulin requirement is recommended by some health care professionals instead of omitting a meal.

5.6.3 Estimating and verifying insulin boluses

Insulin sensitivity decreases with age, especially after the start of puberty. The diurnal variation of insulin sensitivity may be less pronounced in preschool children, as discussed previously. To estimate correction boluses, 100 is divided by the TDD on CSII. Carbohydrate counting (including the estimation of the effect of protein and fat) is strongly recommended for all patients with diabetes. To estimate meal boluses, 300 is divided by the TDD on CSII in preschool children, and the integer 500 is used in bigger children and afterwards (as for adults, see Chapter 3). Human milk (or milk formula) has an equivalent of 7.5g of carbohydrates per 100g (breast-fed infants can be weighted pre- and post-lactation). Human milk and milk formulae may require up to 1U of insulin per 15g of carbohydrate (considerably more than other food). Some children need 2–3 times the usual amount of insulin for covering breakfast.

Meal boluses are best administered 10min before the meal, except during sick days (possibility of vomiting) and in small children (unpredictable eating), where a 'split-bolus' (20% of the total bolus estimation at the beginning of eating, the rest can be added after the meal corresponding to the amount of ingested/retained food) (Box 5.6).

Box 5.6 Estimating insulin boluses

For a 3-year-old girl (when TDD = 10 units):
- Correction boluses = 100 ÷ TDD = 100 ÷ 10 = 10

(1U of insulin decreases BG by10mmol/L)
- Meal boluses: 300 ÷ TDD = 300 ÷ 10 = 30

(1U of insulin covers 30g of carbohydrate)

For a 14-year-old pubertal boy (when TDD = 48 units):
- Correction boluses: 100 ÷ 48 = 2 approx

(1U of insulin decreases BG by 2mmol/L)
- Meal boluses: 500 ÷ TDD = 500 ÷ 48 = 10

(1U of insulin covers 10g of carbohydrate)

Protein and fat considerably alter the absorption of carbohydrates. Composite boluses (e.g. a 'dual bolus') with an addition for higher protein content are recommended. More frequent administration of boluses is associated with better metabolic control. Small tables with pre-calculated boluses for meals and corrections are helpful.

An integrated bolus calculator with preset insulin sensitivities, insulin-to-carbohydrate ratios, and a memory for previously injected boluses (so called 'insulin-on-board'), facilitates bolus estimations, reduces the possibility of 'over-bolusing', and the possibility of an error. Patients may be asked to measure the BG every hour for up to 5hr after a meal to verify the amount and distribution of insulin in a bolus. A CGM device can be conveniently used for the same purpose.

5.7 **Management of hypoglycaemia and DKA**

The BG target range is 4–8mmol/L with a postprandial target <10mmol/L for all age groups (Box 5.7).

Box 5.7 Management of hypoglycaemia on CSII (BG < 3.5) mmol/l)

- Stop the insulin pump for 30min
- Eat 5g of simple carbohydrates (sugar) per 10kg of body weight, to a maximum of 20g
- Measure BG after 15min
  - if still <3.5mmol/L, repeat carbohydrate ingestion
- Eat complex carbohydrate when appropriate (do not overeat!)
- Plan to prevent hypoglycaemia

Measuring urinary or blood ketones is advised when the BG >15mmol/L. It is prudent to verify insulin pump functioning. When catheter or tubing occlusion is suspected, the insulin bolus can be administered with an insulin pen injector and the catheter replaced. In the case of developing DKA, an insulin bolus of 0.1U/kg body weight every hour until the BG falls >10% or <15mmol/L is recommended, plus sufficient oral fluid intake. A health care professional may be contacted.

5.8 Management of activity and exercise

Unpredictable physical activity in toddlers and children is challenging for parents and secondary caregivers. Careful observation of the child helps determine the level of activity. When above average, a 'temporary basal' rate 30%–50% lower than usual can be set on several insulin pump models.

Regular physical activity and sport is highly desirable. BG levels between 5 and 15mmol/L and disconnection from the pump is routinely recommended before strenuous play or exercise. Children can remain disconnected from the pump for up to 1 hour and adolescents for a maximum of 2 hours with a BG check during the activity. A period (4–8 hours) of 'temporary basal' rate 50%–70% lower than usual may be required following prolonged and/or exhausting exercise to prevent hypoglycaemia.

Additional carbohydrate intake is not routinely advised for regular physical activity or sport, unless maintaining zero or positive energy balance is desired. Additional 10–20g of carbohydrate per hour is usually needed for above-average physical activity. Meal boluses after exercise can be reduced by 30%–70%, depending on the activity.

A considerable number of adolescents participate in competitive sports. Individual insulin and meal plans for training and competitions help maintaining good glycaemic control and best sports results.

5.9 Management of sick days

Insulin requirements are generally elevated during sickness. A 20%–50% increase in the basal rate throughout the day is recommended. A separate preset basal rate can be planned for sick days. Meal and correction boluses requirements are also 20%–70% higher during illness. If a child refuses eating or vomits, slightly sweetened fluids can be offered (15–25g of sugar per litre). BG and ketones need to be measured frequently. A health care professional needs to be contacted if DKA is suspected and/or the fluid intake is compromised.

5.10 Managing infusion set insertion and infusion sites

Meticulous skin hygiene is paramount. Insertion is best performed with commercial inserters. Anaesthetising creams (e.g. Emla®) may considerably alleviate pain. Insertion sites can be problematic in infants and toddlers due to limited space and often sparse subcutaneous tissue (Figure 5.1). The area under diapers is more prone to skin maceration and infection. The area above the triceps on the upper arm is a popular insertion site in infants, toddlers, and adolescents (Figure 5.2). The abdominal area is rarely utilized in preschool children. Catheters function from 1.5 to 3 days in infants and children and may last more than 5 days in some adolescents. Several cosmetic creams for skin care may be used (tea tree cream or similar). Antibiotic creams are prescribed in cases of superficial skin infection. Exceptionally, skin incision and/or systemic antibiotics are necessary for infections of subcutaneous tissue.

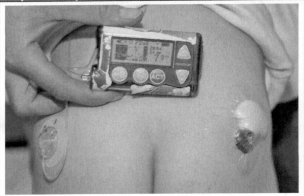

Figure 5.1 Insertion sites of insulin catheter (left) and subcutaneous glucose sensor with transmitter (right) in a 2.5-year-old boy

Current glucose value and a graphical representation of previous 24 hour glucose values are visible on the insulin pump screen.

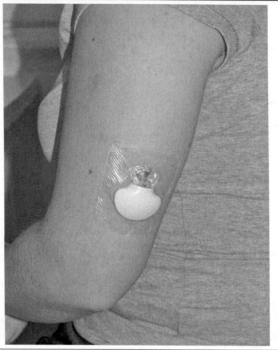

Figure 5.2 Insertion site of a subcutaneous glucose sensor with transmitter on the upper arm in an adolescent

5.11 Educating the social environment of the child and adolescent

CSII may increase the general visibility of diabetes and thus compromise the self-image of children and especially adolescents. Problems related to carrying an insulin pump in the peer environment require thorough discussion at CSII initiation. Kindergarten or school personnel can be invited for a short education session on the essential features of the insulin pump and the management of low and high BG levels. Summer camps offer valuable opportunities for peer discussion on social and practical matters related to using an insulin pump.

5.12 **Downloading insulin pumps**

Logbook keeping is notoriously problematic in children and adolescents, with up to 40% of entries fabricated. Electronic records, which are available for several insulin pump models, include data on insulin delivery and also BG values entered into the integrated dose calculator. A download of the insulin pump at the outpatient consultation provides accurate and detailed information on diabetes management and may serve as a valuable educational tool (Figure 5.3). The download, however, deprives the patient of his liberty to divulge only limited information and it is therefore best employed in a constructive setting.

5.13 **Continuous glucose monitoring**

An RCT has recently demonstrated that the use of RT-CGM devices is associated with significantly lower HbA$_{1c}$ in adults and a significant increase in the proportion of children reaching target HbA$_{1c}$ levels. Several centres of paediatric diabetes routinely use RT-CGM with subcutaneous sensors in toddlers and children (Figure 5.1) where lower A1c can be achieved without increasing the risk of hypoglycaemia (Figure 5.3).

All current RT-CGM devices with subcutaneous sensors lag behind the BG by about 15–20 minutes. When RT-CGM changes rapidly, a considerable difference (up to 3.5mmol/L) is observed between the RT-CGM measurement and the displayed subcutaneous 'real-time' glucose concentration, which often puzzles patients, their families, and health care professionals. Patients and their families need detailed training provided by a diabetes team well acquainted with the technology in order to understand the lag between the subcutaneous and BG concentration and to make use of RT-CGM for predicting glucose trends. When the BG is higher than the one displayed by the RT-CGM device it means that the BG concentration is increasing rapidly. The RT-CGM device will display an upward trend indicator (and alarm) in due course. Patients can be trained to react to the observed difference and prevent further increases in BG even before the upward trend is recognized by the RT-CGM device. Conversely, when the BG is lower than the one displayed by the RT-CGM device, hypoglycaemia may be imminent and timely intervention may prevent it. Recognizing glucose trends and intervening in a timely and balanced manner brings the ultimate benefits of RT-CGM devices.

Over-reaction and miss-reaction on the information provided by a RT-CGM device can worsen metabolic control and may potentially be dangerous. Cases of insulin overdosing have been observed in routine clinical practice because of over-reaction to hyperglycaemia. In addition to thorough education of patients and caregivers, the use of integrated bolus calculators helps in preventing over- and miss-reactions.

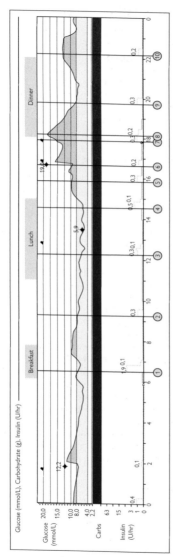

Figure 5.3 A part of the insulin pump and CGM download representing a single day of a 2.5-year-old boy. Black bells represent alarms. Upper line represents glucose levels from the CGM. Values close to this line represent BG measured by a hand BG meter. Lower line represents insulin infusion. The amount of insulin for each bolus is marked above the respective rectangle. Note multiple composite and 'split' boluses. Note how alarms prompted parents to intervene by adding boluses and thus reducing the level and duration of hyperglycaemia. No hypoglycaemia was recorded throughout the day.

5.14 **Closed-loop insulin delivery in children and adolescents**

Ongoing clinical research with fully automated and hybrid insulin delivery systems raises hope in every young patient with diabetes for a careless and limitless life with the disease (see Chapter 9). Insulin pumps that automatically stop delivering insulin when a patient does not respond to the hypoglycaemia alarm of an integrated CGM device have already been approved for clinical use by health care authorities. However bright the future of diabetes technology might be, we currently remain with the tedious task of continuous education and meticulous self-monitoring in order to accomplish optimal metabolic control with the help of CSII and CGM.

References

Battelino T and Bolinder J (2008). Clinical use of real-time continuous glucose monitoring. *Curr Diabetes Rev*, **4**, 218–22.

Campbell F (2008). The pros and cons of continuous subcutaneous insulin infusion (CSII) therapy in the paediatric population and practical considerations when choosing and initiating CSII in children. *British Journal of Diabetes & Vascular Disease*, **8**(Suppl 1), S6–10.

Conwell LS, Pope E, Artiles AM, Mohanta A, Daneman A, and Daneman D (2008). Dermatological complications of continuous subcutaneous insulin infusion in children and adolescents. *The Journal of Pediatrics*, **152**(5), 622–8.

Danne T, von Schütz W, Lange K, Nestoris C, Datz N, and Kordonouri O (2006). Current practice of insulin pump therapy in children and adolescents–the Hannover recipe. *Pediatric Diabetes*, **7**(Suppl 4), 25–31.

Danne T, Battelino T, Jarosz-Chobot P *et al.* and PedPump Study Group. (2008). Establishing glycaemic control with continuous subcutaneous insulin infusion in children and adolescents with type 1 diabetes: experience of the PedPump Study in 17 countries. *Diabetologia*, **51**, 1594–601.

Deiss D, Bolinder J, Riveline JP, *et al.* (2006). Improved glycemic control in poorly controlled patients with type 1 diabetes using real-time continuous glucose monitoring. *Diabetes Care*, **29**, 2730–2.

Diabetes Research in Children Network (DirecNet) Study Group. Tsalikian E, Kollman C, Tamborlane W.B *et al.* (2006). Prevention of hypoglycemia during exercise in children with type 1 diabetes by suspending basal insulin. *Diabetes Care*, **29**, 2200–4.

Jakisch BI, Wagner VM, Heidtmann B *et al.* German/Austrian DPV Initiative and Working Group for Paediatric Pump Therapy (2008). Comparison of continuous subcutaneous insulin infusion (CSII) and multiple daily injections (MDI) in paediatric Type 1 diabetes: a multicentre matched-pair cohort analysis over 3 years. *Diabetes Medicine*, **25**, 80–5.

Juvenile Diabetes Research Foundation Continuous Glucose Monitoring Study Group (2008). Continuous glucose monitoring and intensive treatment of type 1 diabetes. *New England Journal of Medicine*, **359**, 1464–76.

NICE (National Institute for Health and Clinical Excellence) (2008). Continuous subcutaneous insulin infusion for the treatment of diabetes mellitus (Review of technology appraisal guidance 57). NICE Technology Appraisal Guidance 151. Available at: http://www.nice.org.uk/TA151 (Accessed 7 January, 2009).

O'Connell MA, Donath S, O'Neal DN, *et al.* (2009). Glycaemic impact of patient-led use of sensor-guided pump therapy in type 1 diabetes: a randomised controlled trial. *Diabetologia*, **52**, 1250–7.

Opipari-Arrigan L, Fredericks EM, Burkhart N, Dale L, Hodge M, and Foster C (2007). Continuous subcutaneous insulin infusion benefits quality of life in preschool-age children with type 1 diabetes mellitus. *Pediatric Diabetes*, **8**, 377–83.

Pańkowska E, Błazik M, Dziechciarz P, Szypowska A, and Szajewska H (2009). Continuous subcutaneous insulin infusion vs. multiple daily injections in children with type 1 diabetes: a systematic review and meta-analysis of randomized control trials. *Pediatric Diabetes*, **10**, 52–8.

Phillip M, Battelino T, Rodriguez H, Danne T, and Kaufman F (2007). Use of insulin pump therapy in the pediatric age-group: consensus statement from the European Society for Paediatric Endocrinology, the Lawson Wilkins Pediatric Endocrine Society, and the International Society for Pediatric and Adolescent Diabetes, endorsed by the American Diabetes Association and the European Association for the Study of Diabetes. *Diabetes Care*, **30**, 1653–62.

Shalitin S and Phillip M (2008). The use of insulin pump therapy in the pediatric age group. *Hormone Research*, **70**, 14–21.

Szypowska A, Lipka M, Błazik M, Golicka D, Groele L, and Pańkowska E. (2009). Age-dependent basal insulin patterns in children with type 1 diabetes treated with continuous subcutaneous insulin infusion. *Acta Paediatrica*, **98**, 523–6.

Weinzimer SA, Steil GM, Swan KL, Dziura J, Kurtz N, and Tamborlane VV (2008). Fully automated closed-loop insulin delivery versus semiautomated hybrid control in pediatric patients with type 1 diabetes using an artificial pancreas. *Diabetes Care*, **31**, 934–9.

Wiegand S, Raile K, Reinehr T *et al* and DPV-Wiss Study Group. (2008). Daily insulin requirement of children and adolescents with type 1 diabetes: effect of age, gender, body mass index and mode of therapy. *European Journal of Endocrinology*, **158**, 543–9.

Chapter 6

CSII in pregnancy and pre-pregnancy

Peter Hammond

Key points

- Continuous subcutaneous insulin infusion (CSII) should be considered as an alternative to multiple daily insulin injections (MDI), or when an individual on MDI has failed to achieve the tight glycaemic control desirable in diabetic pregnancy (HbA$_{1c}$ <6.1%) without causing problematic hypoglycaemia
- The published literature is very limited in allowing comparison between CSII and MDI in pregnancy, although there is no evidence from randomized controlled trials for any superiority of CSII over MDI
- CSII should be commenced pre-conceptually if possible, since optimized control is desirable before conception takes place
- Intrapartum use of CSII has been shown to be more efficacious at controlling blood glucose levels at the time of delivery and this may reduce rates of neonatal hypoglycaemia
- Combining CSII with continuous glucose monitoring (CGM) may allow better control to be obtained in the later stages of pregnancy and reduce the incidence of macrosomia, but further studies are needed to establish the potential of sensor-augmented pumps in this situation

---

6.1 Impact of diabetes in pregnancy

Pre-gestational diabetes (i.e. people with established diabetes who become pregnant) affects about 1 in 250 pregnancies in the United Kingdom. In addition, up to 4% of pregnancies are affected by glucose intolerance, usually transient and developing in later pregnancy, commonly termed 'gestational diabetes'. Pregnancy in women with diabetes is associated with the increased risks of adverse outcomes for both the woman and the fetus. Glucose is transferred from maternal to fetal circulation by a process of facilitated diffusion. If fetal glucose levels remain normal, then there is no requirement for fetal insulin secretion to control fetal blood glucose, but if the levels become elevated the fetal pancreas starts to produce insulin. Insulin acts as a growth factor for fetal tissues, and fetal hyperinsulinaemia results in the increased growth of insulin-sensitive tissues, increased deposition of adipose tissue, accelerated skeletal maturation, increased hepatic glycogen content, delayed pulmonary maturation due to impaired surfactant production, a delayed switch from fetal haemoglobin (HbF) to HbA, and polycythaemia due to increased erythropoietin production.

In early pregnancy, increased glucose disposal in the fasting state, due to diffusion across the materno-fetal barrier, increases maternal susceptibility to hypoglycaemia. At the same time, due to fetal reliance on glucose for fuel, the mother relies more on ketogenesis to provide fuel substrate, and this increases the risk of developing ketoacidosis. As pregnancy progresses, maternal insulin resistance increases to augment nutrient availability and so there is a need for increasing insulin doses to maintain normal blood glucose levels.

Poor glycaemic control at the time of conception and in early pregnancy is associated with an increased risk of miscarriage and congenital malformation. There is a clear relationship between worsening glycaemic control and spontaneous abortion rates, with similar rates to the non-diabetic pregnant population if women with diabetes have a normal HbA_{1c} at conception, increasing to almost 40% if HbA_{1c} is greater than 9.5% at this time.

Table 6.1 Congenital anomalies associated with diabetes	
Anomaly	Incident ratio (vs. background)
Caudal regression	252
CNS defects	2–10
Anencephaly	3
Cardiac malformations	4
Duodenal and anal/rectal atresia	4
Renal anomalies	5
Agenesis	6
Cystic kidney	4
Duplex ureter	23
Situs inversus	84

In the Confidential Enquiry into Maternal and Child Health (CEMACH) survey from 2002 to 2003 in England, Wales, and Northern Ireland, 3,808 pregnancies in women with type 1 and type 2 diabetes were studied and the rate of congenital malformation was 41.8 per 1,000 live births. There is a particularly high risk of cardiac, renal, and neural tube anomalies and duodenal atresia, whilst caudal regression is almost always associated with maternal diabetes (Table 6.1). Poor glycaemic control through pregnancy is associated with increased rates of stillbirth and perinatal mortality, and in the CEMACH survey the risks were as great for those women with type 2 diabetes as those with type 1 diabetes. Compared with the background population, stillbirth rates were increased 4.7-fold and perinatal mortality by 3.7-fold.

Maternal hyperglycaemia and the consequent fetal hyperinsulinaemia result in an increased incidence of macrosomia (birth weight >4kg); neonatal hypoglycaemia, respiratory distress, and jaundice; and birth trauma, particularly related to caesarean section. There is conflicting evidence relating improved maternal glycaemic control with reduction in these adverse outcomes, and, in particular, tight glycaemic control has not been shown to consistently reduce rates of macrosomia. The excess fetal growth and related neonatal morbidities result in higher caesarean section rates in women with diabetes, as many as two-thirds of these women being delivered in this way, and there is a high rate of admission to neonatal special care units.

In women with diabetes-related complications, pregnancy may have an adverse effect on the progression of complications. Retinopathy may worsen, although this may in part be due to increased blood flow related to high oestrogen levels, and the deterioration often reverses completely following the pregnancy. In the Diabetes Control and Complications Trial (DCCT), those women in the intensively treated arm who conceived were less likely to experience worsening retinopathy than those women on conventional insulin therapy (either once or twice daily insulin), despite the fact that the majority of the latter group transferred to an intensive regimen before or during pregnancy.

There is conflicting evidence regarding progression of nephropathy in relation to pregnancy. In those with mild to moderate nephropathy, there is probably no long-term impact, but in women with a serum creatinine >177µmol/L at conception, there was a 33% risk of accelerated nephropathy, compared with a 2% risk in those with lesser elevations. However, there is often a significant increase in proteinuria in the second half or pregnancy, even in those with only microalbuminuria at the outset. Women with diabetes are more likely to develop pre-eclampsia, particularly if they have hypertension or nephropathy.

6.2 **Intensified insulin therapy in pregnancy**

In order to improve maternal and fetal outcomes, tight glycaemic targets have been recommended for women with diabetes both pre-conceptually and throughout pregnancy. The UK National Institute for Health and Clinical Excellence (NICE) has advised aiming for fasting/preprandial blood glucose levels between 3.5 and 5.9mmol/L, and less than 7.8mmol/L 1 hour post-prandially, and an HbA$_{1c}$ <6.1% pre-conceptually and in the first trimester. NICE does not recommend routine measurement of HbA$_{1c}$ during the later stages of pregnancy.

There is a general consensus that women with type 1 diabetes need an intensified insulin regimen in order to achieve adequate glycaemic control in pregnancy, and many women with type 2 diabetes requiring insulin will also need such regimens. NICE has advised that continuous subcutaneous insulin infusion (CSII) should be considered when adequate glycaemic control cannot be attained because of disabling hypoglycaemia.

In the DCCT, there were 270 pregnancies, exactly half in the intensive and half in conventional treatment groups, although 64 out of 86 women who contributed the 135 pregnancies in the conventional treatment group had switched to intensive treatment pre-conceptually. There was a significant difference in HbA$_{1c}$ between those in the intensive and conventional treatment groups at conception (7.4% vs. 8.1%), and this translated into differences in congenital malformation rates, with eight in the conventional treatment group and one in the intensive treatment group. However, the mean HbA$_{1c}$ during pregnancy was the same in both groups (6.6%).

The options for intensified insulin therapy, as they were in DCCT, are either multiple daily insulin injections (MDI) or CSII via an insulin pump. There is evidence for the superiority of intensive insulin regimens over conventional regimens in terms of glycaemic control, pregnancy complications, rates of spontaneous abortion, fetal outcomes, and neonatal morbidity, including the data from those women enrolled in DCCT who became pregnant.

However, intensified insulin regimens are often associated with a high frequency of hypoglycaemia, particularly in the first trimester, with as many as 40% of women experiencing severe hypoglycaemia, often at night.

6.3 **Insulin pump therapy and pregnancy**

6.3.1 **HbA$_{1c}$ and hypoglycaemia: MDI vs. CSII**

CSII might be expected to have advantages over MDI for both women with diabetes who are planning pregnancy, and for those who are pregnant. Studies in non-pregnant individuals with type 1 diabetes have shown that it is easier using CSII than MDI to achieve tight glycaemic control with reduced rates of severe hypoglycaemia (Chapter 2). Thus, it should be easier for women to achieve the HbA$_{1c}$ target <6.1% using CSII, and any reduction in the risk of hypoglycaemia would be particularly beneficial in the first trimester, when hypoglycaemia is an especially common problem. In later pregnancy, when spikes in maternal glucose could lead to fetal hyperinsulinaemia, the reduction in glucose fluctuations seen in non-pregnant CSII users (Chapter 2) might reduce macrosomia and neonatal morbidity, including hypoglycaemia.

Unfortunately, whilst CSII use by women with diabetes during prepregnancy and pregnancy itself has theoretical benefits there remains a very limited body of evidence concerning this treatment in pregnancy. Most of the literature concerning pump therapy in pregnancy dates from the 1980s, and these studies with early pumps did not demonstrate any superiority of CSII over MDI in terms of glycaemic control or pregnancy-related outcomes; the studies were largely case-control and involved at most tens of patients. Recent meta-analyses of randomized controlled trials (RCTs) of pump therapy during pregnancy have only identified studies fulfilling criteria for inclusion dating from 1993 or earlier.

Given that pump therapy has been reported to be superior to MDI in terms of glycaemic control in non-pregnant individuals in both RCTs and observational studies, it would be expected that this is true for women using pump therapy pre-conceptually. Few studies have compared pre-conceptual control and control during pregnancy for MDI and CSII, and where data are available no significant differences have been demonstrated. However, control does tend to improve in women switching from MDI to CSII.

During pregnancy, glycaemic control tends to improve irrespective of the mode of insulin administration, and therefore it is likely to be more difficult to demonstrate superiority of CSII over MDI during pregnancy. Furthermore, HbA$_{1c}$ may not be as reliable an indicator of control in later pregnancy as it falls in the normal pregnant population due to factors such as a shorter red cell half-life during pregnancy. Studies reporting the effect of CSII compared to MDI on HbA$_{1c}$ through pregnancy, either the mean HbA$_{1c}$ for the whole pregnancy or for different trimesters, consistently show no benefit of CSII over MDI. However, this may be confounded by the selection of women for CSII.

In most observational studies, which comprise almost all of the recent literature and contribute far more cases than the few early RCTs, women are generally switched to CSII when they have problems with control, either an inability to achieve target HbA$_{1c}$, or a high frequency of severe hypoglycaemia. In many cases, the women starting pump therapy have a higher White's classification, an indicator of the prevalence of pre-existing complications and the risk of pregnancy complications. A number of authors have concluded that using CSII in pregnancy allows the achievement of glycaemic control in more women with more complicated and difficult diabetes.

Whilst differences in HbA_{1c} have not been observed, a small number of early studies of pump use in pregnancy did suggest that pumps were associated with a reduction in mean blood glucose, when compared with MDI, and more consistently a reduction in blood glucose excursions. Furthermore, most studies report that CSII usage in pregnancy is associated with less hypoglycaemia, and where CSII has been started because of severe hypoglycaemia, this problem is virtually abolished.

One study has reported the use of CSII in pregnant women with type 2 diabetes or gestational diabetes who were switched to CSII when they required more than 100 units for a single insulin dose by injection. This study demonstrated that good glycaemic control could be achieved in this group of patients without hypoglycaemia.

6.3.2 **Intrapartum glycaemic control**

One study specifically considered the efficacy of CSII in controlling blood glucose levels in the intrapartum period. Women using MDI are almost always switched to intravenous insulin infusion during this stage of pregnancy, but women on CSII have the option to continue using it. There is evidence that CSII is more effective at normalizing blood glucose levels in the intrapartum period than intravenous insulin and that this can reduce the rates of neonatal hypoglycaemia and fetal distress. Whilst other studies have failed to show any impact of pump therapy on neonatal morbidities, including hypoglycaemia, they do not report how blood glucose levels are controlled during labour, and whether women using CSII at the time are switched to intravenous insulin.

6.3.3 **Pregnancy outcomes: MDI vs. CSII**

Observational studies comparing CSII to MDI do not show any superiority of CSII in terms of pregnancy outcomes, insulin requirements, maternal weight gain, maternal or fetal complications, and neonatal morbidity. In particular, CSII does not appear to reduce macrosomia, and there is no difference between CSII and MDI users in terms of large- or small-for-gestational-age babies.

A recent study in pregnant women using either MDI or CSII has shown that frequent use of continuous glucose monitoring during pregnancy can significantly improve HbA_{1c} in the third trimester and reduce rates of macrosomia, compared to women using conventional self-monitoring of blood glucose. It is possible that by using the latest pump technology, which combines pumps with real-time glucose sensors, a greater impact will be seen in terms of improved glycaemic control and reduced rates of macrosomia.

There has been one RCT specifically looking at the progression of retinopathy in pregnancy, which showed no difference between CSII and MDI, but cautioned that two patients who had had very rapid correction of poor glycaemic control had suffered an acute ischaemic retinopathy, which subsequently resolved. It should be noted, however, that DCCT showed that the risk of progression was less in the pregnant women from the intensive treatment arm than those in the conventional treatment arm.

6.3.4 Treatment satisfaction

Despite the apparent lack of superiority of pump therapy over MDI, women who use CSII during pregnancy report high satisfaction with its flexibility, prefer it to MDI, and almost all want to continue using it postpartum and in future pregnancies. There is evidence that women who continue to use CSII postpartum have significantly improved glycaemic control in the months postpartum compared to those using MDI.

6.4 Local experience of CSII in pregnancy and diabetes

In Harrogate, our experience of using CSII in pregnancy contrasts with most of the published literature. We audited 73 pregnancies in diabetes between 1999 and 2007. All women were offered the option of going onto CSII pre-conceptually or at the first presentation in pregnancy. Thirty-nine women were on CSII (nine having switched in early pregnancy), compared to thirty-four women on MDI. HbA$_{1c}$ was significantly lower in the CSII group pre-conceptually (7.3 ± 1.2% vs. 8.2 ± 2.0%) and in the first trimester (6.9 ± 1.1 % vs. 7.7 ± 1.7%). There was no statistical difference in HbA$_{1c}$ in the second or third trimester, but women on CSII experienced significantly reduced rates of hypoglycaemia. CSII users had lower intrapartum blood glucose concentrations, associated with less neonatal hypoglycaemia, compared to those women on MDI who converted to intravenous insulin infusion during labour. Women using CSII had lower weight gain, lower insulin requirements, and maintained a better HbA$_{1c}$ postpartum.

6.5 **Practicalities of using insulin pump therapy in diabetic pregnancy**

There are a number of specific issues that need to be taken into consideration:

- Try to start CSII pre-conceptually, as there is less pressure to achieve immediate improvement in control or reduction in hypoglycaemia frequency, and control should be optimized before conception to reduce the risk of miscarriage and malformation.
- If pump therapy is started during pregnancy, use an initial total daily insulin dose which is 85% of the total daily dose on MDI if blood glucose levels are high, or 80% if hypoglycaemia is a problem. In this way, CSII can be safely initiated in the first trimester without risking worsening control.
- Whilst increments in basal insulin rates tend to be of the order of 0.1–0.2 units/hour in non-pregnancy and the first trimester, in the later stages of pregnancy women may need much greater increments—of the order of 0.3–0.6 units/hour, and they may need to significantly increase the insulin to carbohydrate ratio (by 50% to 100%).
- Pregnancy is associated with accelerated ketosis, as maternal fuel substrates change to allow transfer of glucose to the fetus. Thus, pregnant women with diabetes are at greater risk of ketoacidosis. This has been reported in a couple of cases as a result of pump failure, although in general there does not appear to be an increased risk of diabetic ketoacidosis associated with CSII compared to MDI (Chapter 3). To reduce this risk, we advise women using pumps to check for ketones if blood glucose levels are greater than 10mmol/L, and to changes infusion sets every 2 days.
- Site selection and skin irritation can become a problem in the latter stages as the abdomen expands and abdominal skin tautens. This can be ameliorated by moving sites laterally and posteriorly, and changing infusion sets more frequently.
- Once labour commences, continue using the pump, giving a bolus dose if blood glucose levels increase above 7mmol/L, but changing to intravenous insulin if elevated glucose levels fail to respond. Preset a temporary basal rate to 50% of the term dosage if the pre-pregnancy basal rate is not known. If the woman is breastfeeding, the basal rate may need reducing by a further 10%–20%.

Suggested reading

CEMACH (Confidential Enquiry into Maternal and Child Health (2005). Pregnancy in women with type 1 and type 2 diabetes. CEMACH, London, pp. 76. vailable at: http://www.cemach.org.uk/getattachment/8940bb02-7d42-4067-9aed-92bbecd144ea/Pregnancy-in-women-with-type-1-and-type-2-diabetes.aspx.

Chen R, Ben-Haroush A, Weissman-Brenner A *et al.* (2007). Level of glycemic control and pregnancy outcome in type 1 diabetes: a comparison between multiple daily insulin injections and continuous subcutaneous insulin infusions. *American Journal of Obstetrics and Gynecology*, **197**, 404–6.

Gabbe SG, Holing E, Temple P *et al.* (2000). Benefits, risks, costs and patient satisfaction associated with insulin pump therapy for the pregnancy complicated by type 1 diabetes. *American Journal of Obstetrics and Gynecology*, **182**, 1283–91.

Mukhopadhyay A, Farrell T, Fraser RB *et al.* (2007) Continuous subcutaneous insulin infusion vs. intensive conventional insulin therapy in pregnant diabetic women: a systematic review and metaanalysis of randomized, controlled trials. *American Journal of Obstetrics and Gynecology*, **197**, 447–56.

The Diabetes Control and Complications Trial Research Group (1996). Pregnancy outcomes in the Diabetes Control and Complications Trial. *American Journal of Obstetrics and Gynecology*, **174**, 1343–53.

Chapter 7

CSII in type 2 diabetes

Hélène Hanaire

> ### Key points
>
> - Continuous subcutaneous insulin infusion (CSII) seems more effective than multiple daily insulin injections (MDI) in obese insulin-resistant type 2 diabetic patients in poor metabolic control
> - Education of the patient to the adjustment of the treatment is mandatory
> - CSII is feasible and acceptable in the long term in type 2 diabetic patients, and improves quality of life and treatment satisfaction
> - More scientific evaluation is needed to determine more precisely the indications for CSII in type 2 diabetes

Continuous subcutaneous insulin infusion (CSII) is the most flexible and physiological method of insulin delivery currently available. Its superiority over multiple daily insulin injections (MDI) regimens in terms of HbA_{1c} and frequency of severe hypoglycaemia has been well demonstrated in type 1 diabetes (see Chapter 2), but the use of external pumps in type 2 diabetes is a much more recent area of research and remains debatable (Jeitler et al. 2008; Pickup and Renard 2008).

Type 2 diabetes is associated with insulin resistance and a progressive defect in islet β-cell function. As this defect progresses, in most patients the combination of lifestyle changes and oral antidiabetic agents (OADs) fails to maintain long-term optimal diabetes control and insulin treatment has to be implemented. With bedtime insulin injection combined with OADs commonly used as a first insulin regimen, many type 2 diabetic patients eventually require MDI therapy to maintain blood glucose control. However, even if intensive insulin therapy can improve glycaemic control in obese type 2 diabetic patients, it is often at the expense of high insulin doses, which may lead to marked, further weight gain. In the worst cases, patients gain weight and their glycaemic control remains suboptimal, in spite of increasing insulin doses. Regimens with short- and long-acting insulin analogues are not superior to human insulin-based regimens in terms of HbA$_{1c}$ and insulin doses required, although they can result in a trend towards less hypoglycaemia and weight gain. It is, therefore, tempting to consider the potential indication of insulin pump therapy in type 2 diabetes.

7.1 Potential benefits and risks of insulin pump therapy in type 2 diabetes

On the basis of the observations in type 1 diabetic patients on CSII, one might expect several benefits of pump therapy in type 2 diabetes. A large proportion of type 2 diabetic patients are in poor glycaemic control despite an intensified insulin regimen. CSII is expected to improve glycaemic control in these difficult cases, and reduce glycaemic excursions and the frequency of hypoglycaemic events, even if this problem is far less frequent in type 2 than in type 1 diabetes.

Another concern in type 2 diabetes is the need for large insulin doses and the related weight gain. One might also expect with CSII a limitation of these problems, thanks to a more physiological plasma insulin profile. The pumps currently available are small and user-friendly. The use of an insulin pump might alleviate the burden of intensified treatment and MDI and improve quality of life. The risk of ketoacidosis that requires specific attention and teaching in type 1 diabetic patients on pump therapy is marginal in type 2 diabetic patients.

7.2 Evidence base for the effectiveness of CSII vs. MDI in type 2 diabetes (Box 7.1)

Box 7.1 The efficacy of CSII in type 2 diabetes

- In type 2 diabetic patients with moderately elevated HbA$_{1c}$, the intensification of insulin treatment with MDI or CSII is equally effective
- In obese type 2 diabetic patients with high HbA$_{1c}$ levels, CSII is superior to MDI
- Glycaemic variability, quality of life, and treatment satisfaction are improved by CSII
- There is no difference in hypoglycaemia frequency and weight gain between CSII and MDI
- Metformin can be maintained in association with CSII
- Insulin pump therapy is feasible in the long-term in type 2 diabetes

7.2.1 HbA$_{1c}$

Several authors report a positive experience of CSII in small cohorts of severely obese type 2 diabetic patients in poor glycaemic control (HbA$_{1c}$ 10%–12%) in spite of intensified insulin therapy with high insulin dosages (1.5–5.0U/kg) (Pouwels et al. 2003; Nielsen et al. 2005). Interestingly, in these particularly insulin-resistant patients, both HbA$_{1c}$ and insulin requirements decreased (Wainstein 2001).

More recently, four randomized controlled trials have compared the potential benefits of CSII vs. MDI in insulin-requiring type 2 diabetes (Table 7.1). The trial by Raskin et al. (2003) compared CSII with aspart insulin vs. MDI with pre-meal aspart and one or two injections of isophane as basal insulin. The improvement in HbA$_{1c}$ after 24 weeks was similar in the two groups. In older type 2 diabetic patients (mean age 66 years), the trial by Herman et al. (2005) compared CSII with lispro insulin vs. MDI with glargine and lispro. HbA$_{1c}$ decreased significantly and similarly in the two groups, reaching an optimal level after 1 year. In these two studies, most of the patients were receiving insulin at baseline but not in an intensified regimen, and HbA$_{1c}$ levels were moderately elevated (8.2%). Therefore, it was expected that MDI would be more effective than the baseline treatment in these patients. In these populations, CSII is therefore as effective as but not superior to MDI in terms of overall glycaemic control.

Two other studies, each with a cross-over design, showed a significant improvement in glycaemic control with CSII compared to MDI. The trial by Wainstein et al. (2005), conducted in 40 obese type 2 diabetic patients in poor glycaemic control (HbA$_{1c}$ 10.2%), showed the superiority on HbA$_{1c}$ of CSII with lispro insulin vs. MDI with isophane insulin and human regular insulin. The trial by Berthe et al. (2007) included 17 patients in poor glycaemic control treated by two daily injections of premix insulin (isophane 70/human regular 30), who were allocated to either CSII with lispro insulin or premixed insulin given three times daily. Glycaemic control was improved with both treatments, but to a larger extent on CSII. These two studies indicate the benefit of CSII over MDI; however, the MDI regimens used as comparators were not analogue-based basal-bolus regimens.

7.2.2. Glycaemic variability

Three out of the four randomized studies mentioned above showed a superiority of CSII over MDI in terms of glycaemic variability. Pump therapy improved particularly postprandial glycaemic excursions. Continuous glucose monitoring was performed in the last study (Berthe et al. 2007), and showed a reduction with CSII in not only postprandial excursions but also general glucose variability and in the

Table 7.1 RCTs of CSII vs. MDI in type 2 diabetes

	n	Diabetes duration (yr)	Baseline HbA1c (%)	CSII vs. MDI	OAD	Study type, duration	HbA1c (%) CSII vs. MDI	Insulin dose CSII vs. MDI (U/kg or U/d)	Hypo-glycaemia	Weight change (kg)	Quality of life
Raskin 2003	132	12.5	8%	Aspart vs. 1 or 2 NPH + 3 aspart	No	Parallel-group, 6 mo	NS 7.6 ± 1.22 vs. 7.5 ± 1.22	NS 0.7 vs 0.8 U/kg	NS 0.8 ± 1.6/mo vs. 1.2 ± 3.1	NS +1.7 vs. + 0.9	improved p< 0.001
Herman 2005	107	16	8.3%	Lispro vs. glargine + 3 lispro	No	Parallel-group, 12 mo	NS 6.6 ± 0.8 vs. 6.4 ± 0.8	NS 108 ± 63 vs.108 ± 62 U/d	NS 1.08 vs. 1.22/wk	NS +2.1 vs. +2.6	NS
Wainstein 2005	40	NA	10.2%	Lispro vs. 1 NPH + 3 human reg	met-formin	Cross-over, 2 periods of 4.5 mo	p = 0.007	NS	NS	NA	NA
Berthe 2007	17	17	9%	Lispro vs. 3 premix (lispro-NPH 50/50)	No	Cross-over, 2 periods of 3 mo	p<0.03 7.7 ± 0.8 vs. 8.6 ± 1.6	NS 1.0 ± 0.2 vs. 1.2 ± 0.3 U/kg	NS	NA	NA

time spent in hyperglycaemia. Curiously, hyperglycaemia at the end of the night was not better controlled on CSII than on MDI. This could probably be solved by more accurate adjustments of the basal insulin delivery, much easier to perform with a pump than with injections.

7.2.3 Hypoglycaemia

In all these randomized studies, mild hypoglycaemic episodes are reported at the same (low) rate on MDI and on CSII. Severe hypoglycaemic episodes were also reported to occur with both the treatments in two studies out of four trials. There was no significant difference in the number of patients experiencing severe hypoglycaemia or the number of severe hypoglycaemic events between MDI and CSII. Hypoglycaemia is far less frequent in type 2 diabetes than in type 1. However, recent intervention trials (ACCORD and VADT) designed to evaluate the impact of glucose control on cardiovascular events have focused concern on the frequency and potential danger carried by severe hypoglycaemic episodes. Therefore, particular attention has to be paid to the risk of hypoglycaemia when choosing an intensified insulin regimen.

7.2.4 Insulin dosages and weight

Insulin dosages increased slightly and similarly with both MDI and CSII in all the studies, reaching roughly 1U/kg. There was no difference between CSII and MDI in weight gain, which was moderate and parallel to the improvement in HbA_{1c}. Metformin was used with insulin in only one of the four studies. The insulin sparing effect of metformin and its favourable impact on weight gain deserve being considered not only at the onset of insulin therapy, but also in combination with intensified insulin therapy.

7.2.5 Long-term results

All the above studies were of short duration. In another trial, 59 patients on MDI with poor glycaemic control were switched to CSII and followed for 3 years (Labrousse-Lhermine et al. 2007). The beneficial effects of pump therapy on HbA_{1c} were maintained in the long term (−1.2% at 3 years). Metformin treatment was used with intensive insulin therapy throughout the study. Most of the excess weight reported was gained during the first year of treatment. These results suggest that routine pump therapy in patients with type 2 diabetes, especially those with chronically inadequate glycaemic control, is both feasible and effective in the long term.

7.2.6 **Treatment tolerance**

Infusion site and technical problems occurred with both treatments in the studies. None of them resulted in acute metabolic problems or required hospitalization. Type 2 diabetic patients do not have a full deficit in insulin secretion; therefore, they are not exposed to the risk of ketoacidosis in the event of interruption of the insulin infusion. For this reason, insulin pump therapy might be easier to manage safely in type 2 diabetes.

7.2.7. **Patient satisfaction and quality of life**

Patient satisfaction and quality of life were improved in all the studies. It was particularly well documented in the study by Raskin *et al.* (2003) (Figure 7.1). The CSII patients had significantly greater improvement in overall treatment satisfaction. Ninety-three per cent of the pump-treated subjects favoured the pump for reasons of convenience, flexibility, ease of use, and overall preference. In the long-term study by Labrousse-Lhermine *et al.* (2007), quality of life assessment showed improvement of both objective and subjective criteria, in physical and psychological dimensions. Patients on CSII were better satisfied with their treatment and the impact of the disease decreased. At the end of the 3-year study period, 92% of the patients chose to continue pump therapy, which confirms the good tolerance of the pump and the improvement in quality of life in the long term in patients with type 2 diabetes.

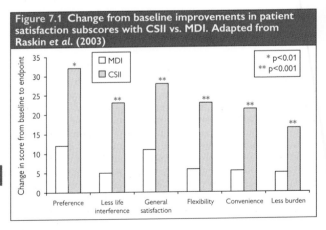

Figure 7.1 **Change from baseline improvements in patient satisfaction subscores with CSII vs. MDI. Adapted from Raskin *et al.* (2003)**

7.3 **Particular indications for insulin pump therapy in type 2 diabetes**

7.3.1 **CSII in pregnant type 2 diabetic patients**

As type 2 diabetes begins earlier nowadays and pregnancies occur later in life, pregnancy in type 2 diabetes is increasing in frequency and importance. Type 2 diabetes in pregnancy is associated with an increased risk of operative delivery and perinatal mortality, which might even be higher than that observed in type 1 diabetes. The control of maternal glucose levels within normal physiological limits has to be obtained as soon as possible, ideally during the preconception period, in order to reduce adverse pregnancy outcomes (malformation, stillbirth, and neonatal death) and very premature delivery. Patients intending to become pregnant or pregnant patients unable to achieve excellent control with optimized insulin injection therapy should be considered for CSII treatment (see Chapter 6). A study conducted in a group of severely insulin-resistant pregnant women with gestational or type 2 diabetes confirmed the safety and efficacy of CSII, particularly in patients requiring large doses of insulin (Simmons et al. 2001).

7.3.2. **Very high insulin requirements**

CSII allows a more predictable subcutaneous insulin absorption rate than MDI with its large volumes injected (Chapter 1). CSII has the theoretical advantages of allowing a smaller volume of administered insulin and the possibility of delivering higher doses. U500 human insulin instead of U100 insulin analogues may be used in the pump reservoir and has proven safe and efficacious in cases of pregnancy and insulin resistance (Knee et al. 2003; Lane et al. 2006).

7.4 **Short-term CSII for uncontrolled diabetes**

Short-term CSII might be considered in type 2 diabetic patients under different circumstances (Hanaire et al. 2008):

- In type 2 diabetic patients with chronic hyperglycaemia and severe insulin resistance, transitory intravenous insulin infusion has been shown to improve blood glucose control. CSII might be an alternative to intravenous insulin therapy and provide, through a wide range of basal rates adjustments, the plasma insulin levels required to overcome the vicious circle of hyperglycaemia and insulin resistance. Pump therapy might be used, for example, in the hospital setting, and/or for a short period of time at home in a well-educated patient. Afterwards, blood glucose control might be achieved with a more simple treatment, assuming that the insulin requirements drop when insulin resistance is lessened.

- Hyperglycaemia or deterioration of glucose control in diabetes due to acute illness is frequently observed in hospitalized patients. It has now been shown to be an independent predictor of morbidity and mortality in critically ill patients. Glycaemic near-normalization in these situations is usually obtained with intravenous intensive insulin, but might also be achieved with CSII (Boullu-Sanchis *et al.* 2006). Continuous insulin infusion is the best way to face unpredictable changes in glycaemia, induced by the severity of the illness, the use of hyperglycaemic drugs such as glucocorticoids, and the variability of food intake.
- When artificial nutrition (enteral or parenteral) is required, continuous insulin infusion is particularly valuable to lessen the large variations of blood glucose which are very difficult to control with discontinuous insulin injections.
- Other transient indications are represented by
  - Severe painful neuropathy
  - Chronic infections, foot ulcers.

7.5 **CSII in newly diagnosed type 2 diabetes**

The decline of β-cell function in type 2 diabetes is affected by glucotoxicity generated by chronic hyperglycaemia. Therefore, the potential benefits of early aggressive intervention with insulin treatment to counteract this negative effect might be considered. Several reports have suggested that short-term intensive insulin therapy with injections or continuous infusion can induce long-term control in type 2 diabetes (Park *et al.* 2003), the predictive factors of success being a shorter history of diabetes, lower postprandial blood glucose levels, and higher body mass index. However, randomized and larger studies would be necessary before concluding that the use of CSII offers real benefits in this indication.

7.6 **Implantable insulin pumps in type 2 diabetes**

Continuous intraperitoneal insulin infusion (CIPII) by means of an implantable pump allows primary insulin absorption by the portal route and results in lower peripheral levels of insulin than with subcutaneous insulin infusion. A randomized controlled trial compared CIPII vs. MDI in insulin-requiring type 2 diabetic patients. The results were similar in terms of HbA$_{1c}$; however, CIPII was superior to MDI for blood glucose fluctuations, mild hypoglycaemia, weight gain, and quality of life (Saudek *et al.* 1996). These results might be explained by the more physiological route of insulin administration.

7.7 **What special groups with type 2 diabetes might benefit from CSII?**

As in type 1 diabetes, patients with type 2 diabetes who cannot achieve optimal glycaemic control with an intensified and well-adjusted MDI regimen might benefit from CSII. In France, insulin pump treatment is reimbursed by the health care system for this indication ('*type 1 or 2 diabetes that cannot be properly controlled through multiple insulin injections*') (Hanaire *et al.* 2008).

The major indication is elevated HbA_{1c}, and the patients who should benefit the most from pump therapy are those whose baseline HbA_{1c} is the highest on MDI (as for type 1 diabetes, see Chapter 2). Pump therapy seems particularly effective, and in some studies superior to MDI, in obese type 2 diabetic patients, and when insulin requirements are large (Nielsen *et al.* 2005; Wainstein *et al.* 2005). The association of metformin may be useful in reducing insulin resistance, insulin requirements, and weight gain. Pregnancy in type 2 diabetes might also be an indication, although the studies conducted in this situation are scarce.

Frequent, mild, or severe hypoglycaemia is a key indication in type 1 diabetes (Chapters 2 and 3), but it is much less frequent in type 2 diabetes and therefore does not represent a usual indication in type 2 diabetes.

In type 2 diabetic patients initiating intensified insulin therapy who have only a moderately elevated HbA_{1c}, insulin pump therapy is as (but not more) effective as MDI, but might improve treatment satisfaction and quality of life. However, for cost reasons, this might not prove sufficient for health care systems to consider these patients as eligible for long-term treatment. It seems reasonable to limit the indications of pump therapy to the patients who have tried and failed to obtain optimal glycaemic control with an intensified insulin injection regimen.

7.8 **Insulin pump therapy in type 2 diabetes in practice**

7.8.1 **Patient selection criteria (Box 7.2)**

Insulin pump therapy can be proposed to patients who present the medical indications for the treatment and who are willing and able to manage it.

Box 7.2 **Selection of patients for CSII in type 2 diabetes**

Medical indications:
- Suboptimal glycaemic control (HbA$_{1c}$ above target) despite intensified insulin injection treatment (MDI) and adequate diabetes management
  - ± wide blood glucose excursions
  - pregnant or planning pregnancy

Ability to manage pump therapy:
- Perform frequent blood glucose monitoring
- Learn the technical components of pump use
- Absence of disability that would impair technical use of the pump
- Comply with recommendations for other components of treatment (diet, exercise, etc.)
- Adjust insulin according to blood glucose monitoring, meals, and different circumstances of daily life
- Comply with safety recommendations and follow up

7.8.2 **Contraindications**

Pump therapy, like any treatment rapidly normalizing glycaemic control, is a contraindication before laser photocoagulation for treatable retinopathy is performed. Severe psychiatric disorders are also a contraindication. Sensory (visual, auditory, touch) or motor impairment/handicap constitute relative contraindications, as in these situations the patient may have difficulties with the technical aspects of pump management and be more dependent on his/her relatives and friends or medical assistance. Pump treatment should not be implemented in case of poor compliance. Patient motivation is mandatory for efficient CSII therapy.

7.8.3 **Education for insulin pump therapy in type 2 diabetes**

Appropriate education for pump therapy is required for type 2 diabetic patients, as for type 1 (Chapter 3). It includes the elements shown in Box 7.3.

7.8.4 **Ongoing evaluation**

An ongoing evaluation of the metabolic results, the compliance, and the satisfaction is necessary, at each visit to the doctor. A complete analysis of benefits, risks, and cost-effectiveness of the treatment has to be performed regularly, in order to confirm or to reconsider the indication of pump therapy in type 2 diabetes.

> **Box 7.3 Main elements of education for CSII in type 2 diabetes**
>
> - Advantages and disadvantages of pump therapy
> - Goals of the treatment
> - Technical management of the pump
> - Blood glucose self-monitoring: frequency, records, interpretation
> - Lifestyle: diet, exercise, weight control
> - How to adjust insulin dosages to achieve blood glucose goals
> - How to adapt treatment in different situations
> - How to deal with hypoglycaemia and hyperglycaemia
> - How to deal with pump-related problems

7.9 **Conclusion**

Pump therapy could be a valuable tool for patients with type 2 diabetes, especially those with chronically inadequate glycaemic control, obesity, and high insulin requirements. It is feasible and well accepted in the long term. Its efficacy requires careful selection of the patients, education, and ongoing evaluation. It seems reasonable to limit the indication to the patients who fail to maintain HbA$_{1c}$ levels at or below target, despite an intensified and accurately adjusted MDI regimen. Stronger evidence is needed of the benefits of pump therapy in type 2 diabetes, and further clinical studies are required to confirm the incontestable indications.

Suggested readings

Berthe E, Lireux B, Coffin C *et al.* (2007). Effectiveness of intensive insulin therapy by multiple daily injections and continuous subcutaneous infusion: a comparison study in type 2 diabetes with conventional insulin regimen failure. *Hormone and Metabolic Research*, **39**, 224–9.

Boullu-Sanchis S, Ortega F, Chabrier G *et al.* (2006). Efficacy of short term continuous subcutaneous insulin lispro versus continuous intravenous regular insulin in poorly controlled, hospitalized, type 2 diabetic patients. *Diabetes & Metabolism*, **32**, 350–7.

Hanaire H, Lassmann-Vague V, Jeandidier N *et al.* (2008). Treatment of diabetes mellitus using an external insulin pump in clinical practice. *Diabetes & Metabolism*, **34**, 401–24.

Herman WH, Ilag LL, Johnson SL *et al.* (2005). A clinical trial of continuous subcutaneous insulin infusion versus multiple daily injections in older adults with type 2 diabetes. *Diabetes Care*, **28**, 1568–73.

Jeitler K, Horvath K, Berghold A et al. (2008). Continuous subcutaneous insulin infusion versus multiple daily insulin injections in patients with diabetes mellitus: systematic review and meta-analysis. *Diabetologia*, **51**, 941–51.

Knee TS, Seidensticker DF, Walton JL, Solberg LM, and Lasseter DH (2003). A novel use of U-500 insulin for continuous subcutaneous insulin infusion in patients with insulin resistance: a case series. *Endocrine Practice*, **9**, 181–6.

Labrousse-Lhermine F, Cazal L, Ruidavets JB, Hanaire H and the Gedec study group (2007). Long-term treatment combining subcutaneous insulin with oral hypoglycemic agents is effective in type 2 diabetes. *Diabetes & Metabolism*.

Lane WS (2006). Use of U-500 regular insulin by continuous subcutaneous insulin infusion in patients with type 2 diabetes and severe insulin resistance. *Endocrine Practice*, **12**, 251–6.

Nielsen S, Kain D, Szudzik E, Garg R, and Dandona P (2005). Use of continuous subcutaneous insulin infusion pump in patients with type 2 diabetes mellitus. *Diabetes Educator*, **31**, 843–8.

Park S and Choi SB (2003). Induction of long-term normoglycemia without medication in Korean type 2 diabetes patients after continuous subcutaneous insulin infusion therapy. *Diabetes/Metabolism Research and Reviews*, **19**, 124–30.

Pickup J and Renard E (2008). Long acting insulin analogs versus insulin pump therapy for the treatment of type 1 and type 2 diabetes. *Diabetes Care*, **31**, S140–5.

Pouwels MJ, Tack CJ, Hermust AR, and Lutterman JA (2003). Treatment with intravenous insulin followed by continuous subcutaneous insulin infusion improves glycaemic control in severely resistant type 2 diabetic patients. *Diabetic Medicine*, **20**, 76–9.

Raskin P, Bode BW, Marcks JB et al. (2003). Continuous subcutaneous insulin infusion and multiple daily injections therapy are equally effective in type 2 diabetes. *Diabetes Care*, **26**, 2598–603.

Saudek CD, Duckworth WC, Giobbie-Hurder A et al. (1996). Implantable insulin pump vs multiple-dose insulin for non insulin-dependent diabetes mellitus: a randomized clinical trial. Department of Veterans Affairs Implantable Insulin Pump Study Group. *JAMA*, **276**, 1322–7.

Simmons D, Thompson CF, Conroy C, and Scott DJ (2001). Use of insulin pumps in pregnancies complicated by type 2 diabetes and gestational diabetes in a multiethnic community. *Diabetes Care*, **24**, 2078–82.

Wainstein J, Metzger M, Wexler ID, Cohen J, and Raz I (2001). The use of continuous insulin delivery systems in severely insulin-resistant patients. *Diabetes Care*, **24**, 1299.

Wainstein J, Metzger M, Boaz M et al. (2005). Insulin pump therapy vs. multiple daily injections in obese type 2 diabetic patients. *Diabetic Medicine*, **22**, 1037–46.

Chapter 8

Real-time continuous glucose monitoring

Howard Wolpert

> ### Key points
>
> - Real-time continuous glucose monitoring (RT-CGM) devices provide detailed information on glucose patterns and trends, and alarms that are triggered by both hyper- and hypoglycaemia
> - Recent trial data indicate that the use of RT-CGM by patients with type 1 diabetes can lead to a reduction in HbA₁c without an associated increase in hypoglycaemia or an actual decrease in hypoglycaemia
> - RT-CGM does not eliminate the need for fingerstick capillary blood glucose measurements. These measurements are required to calibrate the sensor and confirm glucose readings before giving an insulin bolus
> - To use this technology safely and effectively, patients need to have advanced diabetes self-management skills

8.1 Introduction

In the past few years, real-time continuous glucose monitoring (RT-CGM) devices have received regulatory approval for use by ambulatory patients with diabetes. This technology measures the interstitial glucose concentration every 5 minutes, providing the patient with detailed information on glucose patterns and trends, and alarms that are triggered by both hyper- and hypoglycaemia. Current RT-CGM devices approved for long-term clinical use (Abbott Free-Style Navigator, DexCom Seven, and Medtronic Guardian/Paradigm System) have transcutaneous glucose oxidase-based electrochemical sensors that need to be replaced every 3–7 days. These devices are generally less accurate than current fingerstick capillary blood glucose meters; however, this limitation is compensated by the additional information about the rate and direction of changes in the glucose level (Kovatchev et al. 2008). In selected patients, the use of RT-CGM can lead to markedly improved glycaemic control.

8.2 **Randomized controlled trials**

Because RT-CGM is a relatively new technology, only a limited number of randomized controlled trials have been performed. Short-term studies lasting several days have shown that the use of RT-CGM leads to a reduction of both hyper- and hypoglycaemic excursions, with more time in the target glucose range (Garg et al. 2006). The GuardControl trial enrolled 156 adults and children with type 1 diabetes using both pumps and multiple daily injection therapy (Deiss et al. 2006). At 3-month follow up, the group randomized to RT-CGM use had 1.0% ± 1.1% reduction in HbA_{1c} (down from 9.5% ± 1.1% at baseline) compared to 0.4% ± 1.0% reduction in the control group (p = 0.003). At 3 months, 50% of the CGM group had enjoyed HbA_{1c} reductions >1%, compared to 15% in the control group, and 26% had HbA_{1c} reductions >2%, compared to 4% in the control arm. The published report did not indicate the impact of CGM use on hypoglycaemia.

To date, there have been two randomized controlled trials of CGM of 6 months duration. The Star 1 trial enrolled 146 subjects aged 12–72 years with type 1 diabetes treated with continuous sub-cutaneous insulin infusion pumps (Hirsch et al. 2008a). Subjects were randomized to pump therapy with RT-CGM using the Medtronic 722 pump system or to pump therapy with fingerstick self blood glucose monitoring. Baseline HbA_{1c} (8.44% ± 0.70%) declined by a similar degree over the 6-month period in the two study groups (0.71% ± 0.71% in the sensor group vs. 0.56% ± 0.72% in the control group; p = non-significant).

Use of blinded sensors indicated that the control subjects had an increase in the hypoglycaemia area over the curve, whereas in the subjects using RT-CGM the improvement in glycaemic control was not accompanied by a change in biochemical hypoglycaemia (p < 0.0002). Eleven severe hypoglycaemic events occurred in the sensor group and three in the control group (p = 0.04). However, 6 out of the 11 severe hypoglycaemic events in the sensor group occurred while the subjects were not wearing or using the device. In the remaining five events, severe hypoglycaemic episodes were thought to be possibly related to use of the device and the Data Safety Monitoring Board determined that (1) subjects did not respond to alarm warnings of hypoglycaemia; (2) subjects tended to inject multiple boluses of insulin without using the pump bolus calculator, resulting in 'stacking'; or (3) subjects 'blind bolused', that is, they based treatment decisions on sensor glucose readings only, without performing a confirmatory capillary blood glucose measurement. This experience from the Star 1 trial shaped the clinical approach and patient training guidelines followed in the subsequent Juvenile Diabetes Research Foundation CGM trial.

The Juvenile Diabetes Research Foundation CGM trial enrolled 322 patients with type 1 diabetes aged 8–74 years with an HbA_{1c} between 7.0% and 10.0% to either a sensor arm (Abbott Navigator, DexCom Seven, or Medtronic Guardian/722 system) or a control arm that continued with capillary blood glucose monitoring (Juvenile Diabetes Research Foundation Continuous Glucose Monitoring Study Group 2008). A significant between-group difference in change in HbA_{1c} from baseline to 26 weeks was seen in patients ≥25 years old, favouring the CGM group (mean difference in change: −0.53%; $p < 0.001$), but no change was seen in the younger subjects.

Biochemical hypoglycaemia evaluated by CGM did not differ significantly between the two groups. Likewise, there were no significant differences in the incidence of severe hypoglycaemic events between the study groups. In the adult cohort, the frequency of the combined outcome of 26-week HbA_{1c} levels <7.0% plus no severe hypoglycaemic events was 30% in the CGM group and 7% in the control group ($p = 0.0006$). This finding that CGM use leads to a reduction in HbA_{1c} without an associated increase in hypoglycaemia is in direct contrast to most intervention studies in which patients have used intermittent capillary glucose monitoring to guide diabetes self-management.

A separate randomized controlled trial from the Juvenile Diabetes Research Foundation Study Group studied 129 well controlled adults and children with type 1 diabetes who were allocated for 26 weeks to either CGM or conventional monitoring. In this trial, the median time spent in hypoglycaemia (≤60 mg/dl, 3.3 mmol/L) was significantly less for the CGM patients.

8.3 **Practical issues with use of RT-CGM**

To derive full benefit from this technology the patient needs to have advanced diabetes self-management skills, and must have a practical understanding of several key concepts and issues (see Boxes 8.1, 8.2, and 8.3).

8.3.1 **Interstitial glucose measurement and the implications of physiological lag**

Currently available CGM devices measure glucose in the interstitial fluid in the subcutaneous tissue, whereas fingerstick devices measure capillary blood glucose concentrations. When the glucose concentration is changing there is a physiologic lag in the equilibration of glucose between these two compartments. Usually, an increase or decrease in glucose concentration will first be apparent in the blood, followed by the interstitial fluid. This time lag has important implications for the accuracy of continuous sensors and the use of RT-CGM in diabetes self-management.

Since the CGM device is calibrated using fingerstick capillary blood glucose measurements, it is important that the device only be calibrated when the glucose level is relatively stable and there is steady-state equilibration between glucose concentrations in the blood and interstitial fluid compartment (Box 8.1). In practice, this means that calibration measurements should be performed preprandially or at least 3 hours after a bolus. For optimal accuracy, CGM devices should be calibrated at least four times per day (DirecNet Study Group 2006). Patients should also be reminded that blood glucose measurements taken around exercise should NOT be used for calibration. In addition, it is critically important that the patient follow proper procedure in performing glucose measurements to calibrate the continuous monitor. Alternative site measurements for capillary blood testing (e.g. forearm) MUST not be used, and attention must be given to ensuring that fingertips are clean and that the blood glucose monitor is correctly coded according to the manufacturer's instructions.

The physiological time lag can have important implications with regard to detection and treatment of hypoglycaemia. When the glucose is declining, the interstitial glucose generally lags behind blood, and in this situation the actual blood glucose could be quite low even when the interstitial/sensor glucose is normal (Moberg et al. 1997). The practical implication is that, if before driving a motor vehicle, the sensor glucose reading is normal and the glucose level is declining, the patient needs to perform fingerstick glucose measurements. Usually in this situation, the trend graph on the sensor display or rate of change arrows would indicate that the glucose is falling, and this would prompt the patient to check the capillary blood glucose. However, as demonstrated in the study by Wilson et al. (2007), when the glucose is falling rapidly the physiological lag can also lead to underestimation by the rate-of-change indicator of the CGM device. The practical implication of this is that if the sensor indicates that the glucose is both normal and also stable but the patient feels hypoglycaemic or has reason to suspect that the glucose is declining, the patient should disregard the sensor data and do a fingerstick measurement.

Another area where these lag phenomena can be of clinical importance relates to the treatment of hypoglycaemia. Patients who use the sensor to assess whether they are responding to treatment of hypoglycaemia can sometimes end up over-treating the low glucose levels. During the recovery from hypoglycaemia, the increase in the interstitial glucose will often lag behind the blood glucose (Cheyne et al. 2002), and at a time when blood glucose has already normalized the sensor/interstitial glucose may still be in the low range. Patients who rely on the sensor to assess whether their glucose level is improving following ingestion of carbohydrates will mistakenly assume that they need to consume more. The practical implication is that the patient should be informed of the need to perform fingerstick glucose measurements to assess recovery from hypoglycaemia.

Box 8.1 Patient teaching points: calibration DOs and DON'Ts

- Carefully follow the manufacturer's instructions for calibration of the sensor.
- Before calibrating the sensor, check to be sure that the glucose is NOT changing rapidly:
  - There should be NO up or down arrows on the sensor display.
  - If the device does not have rate-of-change indicators, the patient should review the sensor tracing for the previous hour: glucose should have changed by less than 3mmol/L over the previous hour and there should be NO up or down arrows.
- Patients should NOT calibrate:
  - Within 3–4 hours of a meal or an insulin bolus
  - During exercise
  - After recovering from hypoglycaemia.

Box 8.2 Patient teaching points: adjusting bolus doses based on rate-of-change of glucose level (DirecNet Study Group 2008)

- If glucose is increasing 0.056–0.11mmol/L/min, add 10% to calculated food/correction bolus
- If glucose is increasing >0.11mmol/L/min, add 20% to calculated food/correction bolus
- If glucose is decreasing 0.056–0.11mmol/L/min, subtract 10% from calculated food/correction bolus
- If glucose is decreasing >0.11mmol/L/min, subtract 20% from calculated food/correction bolus

---

8.3.2 **Setting glucose alarms**

Alarms for hypo- and hyperglycaemia are an important feature of RT-CGM devices. To ensure that the patient derives maximum benefit from use of the alarms, the alarm thresholds must be individualized (Hirsch et al. 2008b). Table 8.1 outlines some key considerations in optimizing alarm settings.

Setting alarm thresholds is a stepwise process: step 1 entails deciding on initial thresholds when initiating use of the sensor, and step 2 entails reviewing continuous glucose tracings over time to optimize the settings. For patients with hypoglycaemia unawareness or a history of severe hypoglycaemic episodes, the low glucose alarm threshold should be set at 4.5mmol/L or higher. Because of the physiological lag, when the sensor alarm is triggered the blood glucose level will often be lower than the sensor measurement; this is an additional consideration in the setting of the alarm thresholds.

Table 8.1 Trade-offs in setting continuous glucose monitor alarm thresholds	
Set alarms at the 'ideal' level (e.g. low = 4.5mmol/L, high = 10mmol/L)	**Set alarm thresholds more widely** (e.g. low = 3mmol/L, high = 14mmol/L)
Pros: Patient will be warned of most high and low glucose levels	**Pros:** Fewer false alarms Fewer intrusive and irritating alarms Less risk for 'alarm burnout'
Cons: Frequent false alarms Frequent disruption of sleep with associated irritation Increased risk for 'alarm burnout' with related tendency to ignore alarms	**Cons:** Patient will not be warned of all high and low glucose levels

For individuals without a history of problematic hypoglycaemia, the low threshold may initially be set at 3–3.5mmol/L, and the high threshold may be set at ≥14mmol/L. This ensures that while the patient masters the use of the sensor there will be fewer intrusive and irritating alarms, and less risk for 'alarm burnout' (ignoring the alarm). Over time, as the patient uses the information from the sensor to smooth out glucose excursions, the alarm settings can be brought closer to target glucose levels, which may assist with further tightening of glycaemic control.

During follow-up visits, the clinician should establish whether the sensor alarmed whenever the patient's glucose level was low or markedly elevated, and enquire whether the patient was troubled by frequent false alarms. If the patient experiences frequent high glucose levels (especially overnight) and is not being appropriately alerted by the sensor, the high alarm threshold should be reduced. Conversely, if the patient has experienced hypoglycaemic reactions without being alerted, the low alarm threshold may need to be set at a higher threshold.

8.3.3 Minimizing the risk of hypoglycaemia caused by excessive postprandial bolusing

The alarms and trend information provided by CGM devices can be of value in minimizing hypoglycaemia (Box 8.2). However, some patients will over-react to the postprandial glucose spikes identified by the sensor by taking excessive doses of insulin, leading to an increased risk of hypoglycaemia. Reducing this tendency for postprandial over-bolusing is an important focus in the training of the patient using RT-CGM (Wolpert 2008).

Before taking extra insulin to treat postprandial hyperglycaemia, the patient should consider the amount of residual insulin 'on board' from the last pre-meal bolus. Pumps with bolus calculators can assist in making appropriate insulin dose reductions. In addition, knowledge about the glycaemic index of foods is another consideration that can help the patient in deciding whether additional boluses may be required to treat any postprandial hyperglycaemia. With high glycaemic index carbohydrates, a mismatch between the absorption of the carbohydrate and the insulin bolus action will lead to a rapid spike in the glucose levels, but if correction boluses are taken 2–3 hours postprandially there can be an increased risk of hypoglycaemia.

Patients need to be aware that if the sensor tracing or rate-of-change arrow indicates that the glucose level is either rising or falling, they must perform a fingerstick blood glucose measurement before taking insulin. In these situations, 'blind bolusing' without confirmatory fingerstick measurements can be dangerous (Box 8.3).

8.4 **Conclusion**

In selected patients with type 1 diabetes, use of RT-CGM can lead to significant improvements in glucose control. To use this technology safely and effectively, patients need to have advanced diabetes self-management skills and careful guidance from the clinician. Further work is required to identify the psychosocial and other predictors of successful CGM use (Ritholz 2008).

Box 8.3 Patient teaching points: situations where fingerstick capillary glucose MUST be checked

- If the sensor indicates that the glucose is high, before taking an insulin bolus the reading MUST be confirmed with a fingerstick capillary blood glucose measurement.
- Whenever the sensor reading does not seem 'right'.
- If the patient is actually driving a motor vehicle or about to get behind the wheel of a vehicle and the sensor reading is normal, the patient should check if the CGM receiver shows a down arrow, or if the tracing indicates that the glucose level is falling. If the glucose is falling, the patient MUST measure fingerstick blood glucose.
- If, 15min after treatment of a low glucose level, the sensor still indicates that the glucose is low, the patient should check the fingerstick blood glucose level and use this measurement to decide whether to eat more carbohydrate. Reliance on the sensor reading to assess recovery from hypoglycaemia can lead to over-treatment.

References

Cheyne E, Cavan D, and Kerr D (2002). Performance of a continuous glucose monitoring system during controlled hypoglycemia in healthy volunteers. *Diabetes Technology & Therapeutics*, **4**, 607–13.

Deiss D, Bolinder J, Riveline J-P *et al.* (2006). Improved glycemic control in poorly controlled patients with type 1 diabetes using real-time continuous glucose monitoring. *Diabetes Care*, **29**, 2730–2.

DirecNet Study Group (2006). Evaluation of factors affecting CGMS calibration. *Diabetes Technology & Therapeutics*, **8**, 318–25.

DirecNet Study Group (2008). Use of the DirecNet applied treatment algorithm for diabetes management. *Pediatric Diabetes*, **9**, 142–7.

Garg S, Zisser H, Schwartz S *et al.* (2006). Improvement in glycemic excursions with a transcutaneous, real-time continuous glucose sensor. *Diabetes Care*, **29**, 44–50.

Hirsch IB, Abelseth J, Bode BW *et al.* (2008a). Sensor-augmented insulin pump therapy: results of the first randomized treat-to-target study. *Diabetes Technology & Therapeutics*, **10**, 377–83.

Hirsch IB, Armstrong D, Bergenstal RM *et al.* (2008b). Clinical application of emerging sensor technologies in diabetes management: consensus guidelines for continuous glucose monitoring. *Diabetes Technology & Therapeutics*, **10**, 232–4.

Juvenile Diabetes Research Foundation Continuous Glucose Monitoring Study Group, Tamborlane WV, Beck RW, Bode BW *et al.* (2008). Continuous glucose monitoring and intensive treatment of type 1 diabetes. *The New England Journal of Medicine*, **359**, 1464–76.

Juvenile Diabetes Research Foundation Study Group (2009). The effect of continuous glucose monitoring in well-controlled type diabetes. *Diabetes Care*, **32**, 1378–83.

Kovatchev B, Anderson S, Heinemann L, and Clarke W (2008). Comparison of the numerical and clinical accuracy of four continuous glucose monitors. *Diabetes Care*, **31**, 1160–4.

Moberg E, Hagstrom-Toft E, Arner P, and Bolinder J (1997). Protracted glucose fall in subcutaneous adipose tissue and skeletal muscle compared with blood during insulin-induced hypoglycaemia. *Diabetologia*, **40**, 1320–6.

Ritholz M (2008). Is continuous glucose monitoring for everyone? Consideration of psychosocial factors. *Diabetes Spectrum*, **21**, 287–9.

Wilson DM, Beck RW, Tamborlane WV *et al.* and DirecNet Study Group (2007). The accuracy of the FreeStyle Navigator continuous glucose monitoring system in children with type 1 diabetes. *Diabetes Care*, **30**, 59–64.

Wolpert HA (2008). The nuts and bolts of achieving end points with real-time continuous glucose monitoring. *Diabetes Care*, **31**(Suppl 2), S146–9.

Chapter 9

The future of pumps and sensors: research and development

Lutz Heinemann

Key points

- Current pumps are already highly technical and are expected to develop further
- Pumps that receive information from continuous glucose monitoring (CGM) systems are likely to be in increasing use in the coming years. The first type is a version that automatically suspends insulin delivery in the event of hypoglycaemia, the first step towards an artificial pancreas
- A fully closed-loop insulin delivery device with a glucose sensor coupled to a computer-controlled insulin infusion pump is being actively researched. It is a complex problem that may require some years of development. A hybrid system with patient-activated meal-time insulin and closing-the-loop only in the basal state is a likely first development for clinical use
- Smaller, simpler patch pumps with integrated cannulae and novel pumping mechanisms are under development. Some may be used in type 2 diabetes
- Fully implantable insulin pumps have been in the research phase for some decades and, as yet, have significant problems for transfer to widespread routine clinical use

9.1 Evolution of conventional insulin pumps

Pumps that allow infusion of insulin with a variable basal rate and infusion of boluses before meals have come a long way in the past 30–40 years, in numerous development cycles, from systems that weighed several kilograms and were carried around as a backpack to the present small 'high-tech' systems. Today's insulin pumps are easy-to-use in daily life, highly reliable, and offer many different features (see Chapters 1 and 4). Pumps can even be controlled by a remote pager-like device, with no direct handling of the pump. Patients value pumps becoming more discrete in this way, though the absence of regular visual inspection of proper pump functioning may be a downside.

The handful of companies that are already in the market introduce 'improved' pumps every few years. Owing to demanding regulatory hurdles and requirements, developing a truly new insulin pump rather than a variation of an old technology is more expensive and time-demanding than one would first think. Pump developments clearly also depend on the rapidity of technological advances in other areas: lighter batteries with more electrical power, central processors with more calculation power, displays with improved readability (e.g. in colour), and most importantly pump motors of considerably less size. Smart usage of these developments has led to the advanced insulin pumps of today.

Such technological developments are unlikely to have reached a standstill. One can envisage flexible displays with organic light-emitting diodes (LEDs) that cover most of the pump surface, more 'brain' in the pumps due to computer processors with high computational power but reduced power consumption, and smaller batteries with more capacity allowing longer usage without exchange, and the construction of even smaller pumps. It may be possible in the future to speak with the insulin pump, changing basal rates and boluses by voice. The capability to download data is already a feature of some current pumps (see Chapter 4), but one must soon expect automatic downloads for analysis of errors and for expert advice. This could show patients (adolescents might benefit especially) when they have forgotten a bolus, and when they should have measured blood glucose levels more often.

The choice and the number of additional materials and consumables required for pump therapy such as catheters and infusion sets have improved considerably in recent years. For example, usage of different materials for insulin catheters (polyethylene instead of poly-vinylchloride) has improved handling. Usage of catheters which are coloured could enhance visibility of air bubbles. One can envisage further options to meet the needs of different patients and physicians. Another possible development is insulin reservoirs that are not made of glass or clear plastic but more like small flexible plastic bags. Bags that fulfil the stringent requirements for sterility and stability as drug containers have taken some time to develop. The availability of such insulin reservoirs enables construction of insulin pumps of a different shape, particularly ones that are much flatter than conventional pumps. Clearly, such bags require new pumping technologies, since a plunger is not advanced in a syringe-type reservoir. Such pumps must guarantee that insulin is pumped at all times.

The many new technological features and capabilities in pumps which have been introduced or are to be expected may have disadvantages: systems may be so complex that many patients never use all these features in daily practice (Jankovec et al. 2008). Pumps that have both a basic and an advanced user-level may be popular. In addition, some of the new features and pump concepts that work well in the laboratory might fail in the rough conditions of daily life, and rigorous attention to patient needs, capabilities, and everyday practicality will be essential for pump development.

It is sometimes the marketing value that drives the introduction of increased features in consumer devices (as with mobile phones); however, the scientific evidence that such features are of real help or importance for the patient is sometimes missing. For example, modern pumps offer a number of different ways to infuse the meal insulin. Depending on the content of the meal (low or high glycaemic index, fat or protein content), the meal duration, and gastric emptying patterns, it is suggested that different profiles of prandial insulin can be used—immediate, extended, or dual wave (Chapter 4). However, we need to increase the clinical and experimental evidence base for the use of such profiles.

Like other medical device companies, pump manufacturers have hitherto conducted few such studies. In the present era of evidence-based medicine and the critical questioning of health care insurers and national health services about the cost/benefit ratio of insulin pump therapy ('Is a small improvement in glycated haemoglobin along with more flexibility in daily life worth the higher costs?'), it will become critical to demonstrate evidence of value to be eligible for reimbursement or national funding.

With the economical crisis in health care systems around the world and the increasing use of insulin pump therapy (on clinical grounds and as a patient preference), it is not clear who will pay for this therapy option in the future. Payment cannot be confined to the costs of new pumps and consumables per se. Proper usage also requires time from the physician and the diabetes team to explain the device operation and new treatment strategies, to answer questions, download data, and interpret them, and supervise on-going care. Cost-effectiveness analyses to date have not always included such time (Chapter 2) but it must be factored into the costing in the future and probably new payment models developed.

Improved efficacy of insulin pump treatment may be driven by not only new technology but also other options. For example, more rapid and consistent absorption of insulin from the subcutaneous tissue (e.g. after a meal bolus) might be achieved by new formulations of insulin with additives that enhance dissociation into monomers (e.g. VIAject™ insulin, Biodel Inc., USA), by intradermal infusion by means of ultra-short needles (Becton-Dickinson, USA), or by application of heat to the skin above the infusion site (InsuLine, Israel) (Pettis *et al.* 2006; Steiner *et al.* 2008). Also, smarter infusion algorithms might help to establish new steady-state insulin levels after changing the basal rate by employing a priming dose (with an increase in the basal infusion rate) or by stopping the infusion completely for a certain period of time. However, in view of the insulin depot of some units that exists around the needle tip in the subcutaneous tissue, it is possible that such changes in the infusion rate will not have a rapid enough effect (see later).

9.2 Continuous glucose monitoring and insulin pumps

9.2.1 Sensor-augmented and smart pumps

A more recent trend is that the blood glucose meter used by the patients can transfer the reading automatically to the insulin pump. In combination with a bolus calculator, changes to insulin delivery can be made without the need for manual data transfer. This simplifies pump therapy and avoids potential handling errors (while introducing potentially others, see later). However, most patients do not perform more than 4 or 5 capillary blood glucose tests per day and such spot measurements provide only a snap shot of the glucose profile over the day. In contrast, continuous glucose monitoring (CGM) follows all glucose swings during the day and night (Chapter 8). Patients are often shocked to see how variable their glycaemic control is throughout the day, ranging from extreme high levels to unrecognized hypoglycaemia. It is important for patients to understand the differences between capillary blood glucose measurements and glucose monitoring in the interstitial fluid by CGM systems, and close interaction with the diabetes team, and advanced diabetes self-management skills are needed by the patient to make best use of CGM data (Chapter 8).

Pumps are currently available which allow display of CGM data (Paradigm® Real-Time, Medtronic). Glucose readings from the sensor inserted into the abdominal subcutaneous tissue are transferred to the pump by radio-wave frequencies from a small link device connected to the electrode. The pump displays the glucose profile of the last 3 or 12 hours, with the current glucose concentration and an arrow indicating the trend in glucose changes. An audible alarm signals glucose levels which fall below a self-defined low-level limit or increase above a high-level limit. Other companies are expected to bring such sensor-augmented pumps to the market in the coming years.

Glucose trend information allows the pump to be 'smart'. Not only can an alarm be activated, but in a version recently introduced the pump suspends insulin infusion for a short period when low blood glucose levels are detected by the CGM, thus allowing glucose to recover (Buckingham et al. 2008; Dassau et al. 2008). In the future, sensor pumps could alarm a central reporting station at the local hospital or at the treating physician's office in the event of blood glucose remaining in the low range for a prolonged period and its user not responding to the alarm (accompanied by an automatic stop of the insulin infusion, see later). This could be achieved by activating automatically the mobile phone of the user.

In a similar fashion, CGM could temporarily activate an increased insulin infusion rate in pumps if blood glucose levels reach or trend towards hyperglycaemia. However, in view of the delay in subcutaneous insulin absorption, acute changes in pump rates may have limited short-term effects. The next level of smartness for the pump would be to analyse metabolic deteriorations over several days and adjust, for example, the basal rate or bolus delivery to reduce future events (pattern analysis). If an accelerometer is build into the pump, the activity profile of the user could be analysed and insulin delivery rates adjusted appropriately.

Smart pumps could also indicate when it is time for the next meal, recommend a carbohydrate/insulin ratio depending on the time of the day, indicate that a bolus should be delivered but some metabolic activity is remaining from the previous bolus, or that the amount of insulin in the reservoir is coming to an end. Information provided by a CGM device might train the algorithm of bolus 'wizards' according to the real needs of its user. Owing to inter-individual differences in insulin absorption, eating behaviour, digestion, and nutrient absorption, a general algorithm does not always meet individual needs.

If preprandial glycaemia is high, the pump might advise the patient to wait before starting the meal to allow blood glucose levels to decline. Some patients will welcome such advice, whilst others will prefer less automatic instructions. The uptake of these sensor-pump 'advisers' will also depend on the level of teaching of the patient. An informed ('smart') patient with good knowledge of diabetes, insulin pharmacology, and pump technology might prefer to make decisions himself. Those who prefer to transfer or share responsibility for their care may like the information provided. However, sometimes the logic behind current advice systems is obscure. For example, the duration of insulin action is an important component of the bolus calculator for most modern pumps, but it is interesting to see that the times used in the calculators of different pumps differ considerably, even for the same insulin (Chapter 3).

Sensor pumps can also analyse glucose profiles over 24 hours or several days and provide summary measures of control such as indices of glucose variability. It should be possible to provide information on why a hypoglycaemic event has taken place by displaying this part of the glucose profile along with other relevant information such as whether the insulin bolus was too large. Which of these innovations/features are real improvements and which are just gadgets is not easy to judge before clinical evaluation; a feature might be regarded as nonsense for the scientists/clinician but is highly welcomed by the end user.

CGM-pump combinations may become standard in the near future, at least as one pump option, but the higher costs compared to standard injection or infusion therapy are an important consideration. Whilst engineers and computer experts bring their dreams to life with smarter pumps and sensors, 'value' for patients with diabetes must be demonstrated. And without additional teaching and training of patients, technical developments may be of limited worth. At least the clinical efficacy of sensors and sensor pumps is becoming clearer. In adults with type 1 diabetes (but not children or adolescents), it was recently demonstrated in a randomized controlled trial that usage of CGM and insulin pumps (80% of the patients used CSII) lowered HbA$_{1c}$ in comparison to the control group (JDRF, Continuous Glucose Monitoring Study Group 2008). It appears that the more frequently and the longer the CGM system was used the better was the metabolic control. In this study, children and especially adolescents made less use of sensors which was reflected by the absence of significant improvement in HbA$_{1c}$ in this group. This highlights the need for an appropriate teaching and training programme to accompany such technological improvements.

In the United States, reimbursement for CGM is now provided by a number of health care insurers. This is mandatory to ensure that the market will remain attractive for companies developing such systems. Investment to date has been high without much financial return. But health–economic considerations must include factors other than quality of control. Technology-driven avoidance of acute metabolic deteriorations reduces the fear of future hypoglycaemia and tissue complications, enabling patients to improve metabolic control with more confidence. Also, the well-being of the patients most probably will be improved, which allows them to be more productive in their working life. Estimates of cost–benefit ratios therefore depend on many factors, and some are difficult to handle in the models currently applied to these calculations (see Chapter 2).

9.2.2 Glucose sensing in the future

The disadvantages of the currently available CGM systems are the relatively short duration of usability of sensors (up to about 7 days), the pain that is associated with insertion of these minimally invasive needles into the subcutaneous tissue, the risk of infection due to breaking the skin barrier, the limited measurement quality, especially at low blood values, and the fact that glucose changes are monitored in the interstitial fluid and not directly in the blood stream (Chapter 8).

More reliable and affordable sensors are to be expected. A number of companies are developing minimally invasive CGM systems with improved function, using, for example, nanotechnology approaches. Clearly the dream is to have a CGM system like a wristwatch that can monitor changes in glycaemia non-invasively for prolonged periods of time without having the need of breaking the skin barrier. However, despite >30 years of intensive work on non-invasive glucose sensors and the investment of at least one or two billion dollars, no system that allows non-invasive glucose monitoring in daily life with sufficient reliability is available. Despite more or less regular announcements that the 'breakthrough' has been achieved, many scientists are more sceptical than ever that it will be possible to monitor glucose non-invasively. This is particularly so with the near-infrared spectroscopy approach which has been studied most intensively in the past few decades. Probably other approaches, for example, impedance spectroscopy, can be developed to a level that at least allows reliable monitoring of trends in glycaemia (Caduff et al. 2006).

An alternative approach is the total implantation of a glucose sensing device with subsequent non-invasive measurements from outside the body, for example, using fluorescent light (Pickup et al. 2005). Such an implanted sensor might require a run-in period of up to some weeks before it works appropriately, but might then function for several months requiring re-calibration only at long intervals. With these systems, glucose measurements can be discrete or continuous, depending on the technology. So far, none of these approaches has entered extended clinical research and testing. One caveat is that some glucose sensing molecules are toxic and it is unclear whether the regulatory authorities will accept insertion of such implants, even if only tiny amounts are inserted and are well covered.

9.3 Closed-loop insulin delivery: the artificial pancreas

A reliably working CGM system in combination with an insulin pump with sufficient computer power makes the step toward a closed-loop insulin delivery system look like a small one. In reality, this 'technological cure for diabetes' is complex and difficult. It is a dream for patients with diabetes and for diabetologists (Renard 2002; Hovorka 2006).

The first requirement for safe and effective closed-loop diabetes control is a highly reliable CGM system. Currently available systems do not yet meet this need. Glucose information from the CGM is transferred to a control system (which might be a part of the pump) and a computer compares actual and nominal blood glucose values and, according to algorithms, alters insulin infusion to minimize the glycaemic disturbance.

The development of suitable algorithms to match physiology is a complex task. In normal individuals, periods of low, relatively constant insulin secretion during the night and between the meals alternate with periods of rapid and marked increases and then decreases of insulin secretion at mealtimes. Algorithm calculations are usually based only on glucose concentrations, but physiological increases in insulin secretion occur at the mere sight of food, and gastrointestinal functioning after a meal also has an impact on glucose absorption and metabolism.

It is intended that an increase of glycaemia should be restricted in closed-loop systems by increased insulin infusion, but subcutaneously administered insulin is slowly and unpredictably absorbed into the blood and needs time to cause its biological effect. Even the use of fast-acting insulin analogues does little to reduce the lag between glucose sensing and insulin action. Another possibility to reduce lag times is the infusion of insulin into alternative sites where it is absorbed more rapidly. The infusion of insulin into the peritoneum, either by an implanted insulin pump (see below) or via a port with indwelling catheter (Diaport), is an alternative option, though intraperitoneal insulin delivery has been associated with significant problems over the years (omental blocking of the cannulae, abdominal adhesions, peritonitis).

To counteract falls in glycaemia, glucose infusion appears logical. However, subcutaneous glucose administration induces pain and would require a large volume to be stored and pumped. An alternative is the infusion of glucagon to mobilize glucose stored in liver glycogen. This therefore requires dual pumping of insulin and glucagon (El-Khatib et al. 2008).

Several companies are collaborating with academic groups to achieve closed-loop coupling of real-time CGM system with insulin pumps (e.g. Medtronic Inc. with the Paradigm® Real-Time insulin pump), with the intention of eventual commercialization. The impressive efficiency of the algorithms and technology used in such systems was shown in a recent publication with 10 patients with type 1 diabetes (Steil et al. 2006). Though glycaemic control did not match that of healthy subjects, particularly after meals, a general improvement over open-loop delivery was seen.

Complete 'physiological' insulin substitution with an artificial pancreas might not be achievable. Acceptable metabolic control might only be possible with current technology if input is given by the user at meals and other times ('semi-closed loop systems'), that is, information about meals (content and time of intake) is given to the system or the patient activates meal insulin delivery manually, or information about intended physical activity (duration, intensity) is provided to the algorithm (Weinzimer et al. 2008). Closed-loop control during nights is now achievable (when there is a more stable metabolic situation) without intervention by the user (Hovorka et al. 2008).

Everyday life consists of different requests and conditions around which such a system as an artificial pancreas is expected to work error-free. Malfunctions in sensing and system controls which cause too little insulin to be delivered and a small rise in blood glucose might result in only limited immediate problems, but too much insulin might result in substantial acute problems and a significant safety risk. This highlights the problem of liability. Is the patient able to prove that he had this accident because of a malfunction of the closed-loop system, and has the manufacturer to pay the possibly extensive costs of the accident? This problem could perhaps be avoided if patients had to acknowledge every change in insulin infusion rate by pressing a button. Thereby, therapeutic decisions remain with the patient who can evaluate the situation, though this would take away the closed-loop goal of 'forgetting about diabetes'.

9.4 Patch, disposable, and implantable pumps

Current insulin pumps are relatively expensive, complex to use, and require considerable staff and patient training. New pump concepts are needed, such as pumps without catheters, smaller and simpler pumps (say, for infusing a basal rate only), and disposable pumps (Rave et al. 2007; Kapitza et al. 2008). These developments should make insulin pump therapy easier and more affordable.

Handling of the pump catheters and insertion of the needles is most probably the most unwelcome part of pump therapy. Automatic insertion of the needle by a system that is hidden inside the insulin pump is a potential way to overcome these issues (e.g. Omnipod). Avoidance of the catheter and automatic insertion/retraction of the needle are attractive options. Such pumps should also allow usage under all daily life conditions, without any safety risk or discomfort for activities such as showering, swimming, sports, sex, sleeping, and so on. They might also reduce the risk of infection at the needle insertion site or other local skin reactions combined with repeated application of the needle at a given skin site.

Pumps are already fulfilling some of these new engineering expectations, for example, for new catheter design. It is noteworthy that new pump companies also need a substantial sales force and a sound marketing structure, sometimes a big undertaking for a small company. The production costs of insulin pumps have to be much lower than the selling costs in order to cover associated costs such as a 24-hour telephone advice service and the provision of immediate exchange of defective pumps.

Companies that have declared an intention to develop smaller and (probably) cheaper pumps include (in alphabetical order) Debiotech from Switzerland, Danfoss from Denmark, Medipacs from the United States, Medingo Medical Solutions from Israel, Sensile another Swiss company, Starbridge Systems from United Kingdom, and Victoria from Australia. Some of the larger pharmaceutical companies that are also active in the medical device field (e.g. Novo Nordisk) are also working on novel insulin pumps. The technology used in these pumps to infuse insulin differs considerably, from small high-tech mechanical pumps to membrane pumps driven by piezoelectric crystals, to pumps making use of the self-contracting force of elastomers (pressure pumps).

A probable market for such new pumps is type 2 diabetes. Although the evidence base (from randomized controlled trials) for insulin pump treatment in this patient group is weak (Chapter 7), in many of these patients who presently use a long-acting insulin analogue, a 'simple' pump that infuses insulin with a constant basal infusion rate might be sufficient and efficacious (Jeitler et al. 2008). Usage of such 'patch-pumps' might be limited to subgroups in the very heterogeneous type 2 diabetes. Although a small percentage of all people with type 2 diabetes might benefit, in absolute numbers millions of patients could use CSII as a therapeutic option (Parkner 2007).

Some 20 years ago, many assumed that implantation of insulin pumps will be successful, based on several perceived advantages (Renard et al. 2007). From first experiments in animals in the 1970s, a clearly more rapid absorption of intraperitoneal (IP) infused insulin was demonstrated. The implantable pump would be invisible and not mark the person as having diabetes. Owing to insulin transfer via the portal venous system into the liver, peripheral plasma insulin levels are lower than when using the subcutaneous route but more effectively suppress hepatic glucose production. Safety, effectiveness, and reduction of blood glucose variability, associated with long-term usage of implanted insulin pumps, were reported in a series of studies (Saudek et al. 1989).

IP insulin delivery at a lower cost and with higher patient autonomy than with implantable pumps can be achieved with a device such as the DiaPort® system, developed by Roche Diagnostics (Mannheim, Germany). This system includes a port that is implanted in the abdominal wall to which an IP catheter is connected on one side, and an external insulin pump on the other side. Clinical investigations have reported close-to-physiological blood glucose and plasma insulin profiles while using such ports for IP insulin delivery (Hammond *et al.* 2007).

So far, the clinical use of implantable insulin pumps (several hundreds have been implanted) is very limited because of the cost, the limited availability of the insulin delivery devices, the need for special insulin which remains stable at body temperature and the invasiveness of implantation. The costs are related to the device cost itself but also to the man-time cost needed to implant the pump, to refill the pump reservoir with insulin in hospital every 8–12 weeks and to maintain reliable insulin delivery. Despite these issues, several specialist diabetologists strongly believe in the future of this type of insulin pump (Renard *et al.* 2007), but its widespread uptake is generally regarded as uncertain or unlikely.

References

Buckingham B, Cobry E, Clinton P et al. (2008). Preventing hypoglycemia using predictive alarm algorithms and insulin pump suspension. *Diabetes*, **57**(Suppl. 1), A66–7.

Caduff A, Dewarrat F, Talary M, Stalder G, Heinemann L, and Feldman Y (2006). Non-invasive glucose monitoring in patients with diabetes: a novel approach based on impedance spectroscopy. *Biosensors and Bioelectronics*, **15**, 598–604.

Dassau E, Cameron FM, Lee H et al. (2008). Real-time hypoglycemia prediction using continuous glucose monitoring (CGM), a safety net to the artificial pancreas. *Diabetes*, **57**(Suppl. 1), A13.

El-Khatib FH, Jiang J, Damiano ER (2008). Closed-loop blood-glucose control using dual subcutaneous infusion of insulin and glucagon in ambulatory diabetic pig. *Diabetes*, **57**(Suppl. 1), A23.

Hammond P, Liebl A, and Grunder S (2007). International survey of insulin pump users: impact of continuous subcutaneous insulin infusion therapy on glucose control and quality of life. *Primary Care Diabetes*, **1**, 143–6.

Hovorka R (2006). Continuous glucose monitoring and closed-loop systems. *Diabetic Medicine*, **23**, 1–12.

Hovorka R, Acerini CL, Allen J et al. (2008). Overnight sc-sc closed-loop control improves glucose control and reduces risk of hypoglycaemia in children and adolescents with Type 1 diabetes. *Diabetes*, **57**(Suppl. 1), A22.

Jankovec Z et al. (2008). Frequency of available insulin pump functions use by patients with diabetes mellitus. Abstract 112, 1st ATTD Meeting, Prague.

JDRF Continuous Glucose Monitoring Study Group (2008). Continuous glucose monitoring and intensive treatment of Type 1 diabetes. *New England Journal of Medicine*, **359**, 1464–76.

Jeitler K, Horvath K, Berghold A et al. (2008). Continuous subcutaneous insulin infusion versus multiple daily insulin injections in patients with diabetes mellitus: systematic review and meta-analysis. *Diabetologia*, **51**, 941–51.

Kapitza C, Fein S, Heinemann L, Schleusener D, Levesque S, and Strange P (2008). Basal-prandial insulin delivery in type 2 diabetes mellitus via the h-patch™: a novel continuous subcutaneous infusion device. *Journal of Diabetes Science and Technology*, **2**, 40–6.

Parkner T, Laursen T, Chen JW et al. (2007). Overnight versus 24 Hours of continuous subcutaneous insulin infusion as supplement to oral antidiabetic drugs in Type 2 diabetes. *Journal of Diabetes Science and Technology*, **1**, 704–10.

Pettis RJ, Hompesch M, Kapitza C, Harvey NG, Ginsberg B, and Heinemann L (2006). Intra-dermal insulin lispro application with a new microneedle delivery system led to a substantially more rapid insulin absorption than subcutaneous injection. *Diabetes*, **55**(Suppl.1), A26.

Pickup JC, Hussain F, Evans ND, Rolinski OJ, and Birch DJS (2005). Fluorescence-based glucose sensors. *Biosensors and Bioelectronics*, **20**, 2555–65.

Rave K, Heinemann L, and Gravesen P (2007). Pharmacokinetic and pharmacodynamic effects of a sc infusion of insulin Lispro by a disposable basal insulin pump in healthy volunteers. *Diabetes*, (Suppl. 1), A120.

Renard E (2002). Implantable closed-loop glucose-sensing and insulin delivery: the future for insulin pump therapy. *Current Opinion in Pharmacology*, **2**, 708–16.

Renard E, Schaepelynck-Belicar P and on behalf of the EVADIAC group (2007). Implantable insulin pumps. A position statement about their clinical use. *Diabetes & Metabolism*, **33**, 158–66.

Saudek CD, Selam JL, Pitt HA et al. (1989). A preliminary trial of the programmable implantable medication system for insulin delivery. *New England Journal of Medicine*, **321**, 574–9.

Steil GM, Rebrin K, Darwin C, Hariri F, and Saad MF (2006). Feasibility of automating insulin delivery for the treatment of type 1 diabetes. *Diabetes*, **55**, 3344–50.

Steiner SS, Hompesch M, Pohl R, Simms P, Pfützner A, and Heinemann L (2008). A formulation of human insulin with a more rapid onset of action than rapid-acting insulin analogues. *Diabetologia*, **51**, 1602–6.

Weinzimer SA, Steil GM, Swan KL, Dziura J, Kurtz N, and Tamborlane WV (2008). Fully automated closed-loop insulin delivery versus semiautomated hybrid control in pediatric patients with type 1 diabetes using an artificial pancreas. *Diabetes Care*, **31**, 934–9.

Appendix

Useful websites

Insulin pump manufacturers (not all pumps are available in all countries):

Animas—2020 Pump, One Touch Ping
www.animascorp.com

Deltec—Cosmo pump
www.cozmore.com
www.smiths-medical.com

Insulet—Omnipod
http://www.myomnipod.com/

Medtronic-MiniMed—Paradigm pumps
www.minimed.com
www.medtronic-diabetes.co.uk

Nipro—Amigo pump
http://www.niprodiabetes.com

Roche—Accu-Chek Insulin Pumps
www.accu-chek.co.uk
www.accu-chek.com

Sooil—Dana Diabcare IISG
http://www.sooilusa.com

CGM (continuous glucose monitoring) manufacturers (not all CGM systems are available in all countries):

Abbott—FreeStyle Navigator
www.freestylenavigator.com

DexCom—Seven CGM System
www.dexcom.com

Medtronic—MiniMed Paradigm Real-Time CGM, Guardian Real-Time System
www.minimed.com/index.html
www.medtronic-diabetes.co.uk

Patient support groups

INPUT
www.input.me.uk

Insulin pumpers
http://www.insulin-pumpers.org
http://www.insulin-pumpers.org.uk

My Pump
http://www.mypump.co.uk/index.htm

Diabetes and Sport
www.runsweet.com

Diabetes associations and guidance

Diabetes UK
www.diabetes.org.uk

Juvenile Diabetes Research Foundation
www.jdrf.org

American Diabetes Association
www.diabetes.org

NICE
www.nice.org.uk

Index